HEAD
IN THE
GAME

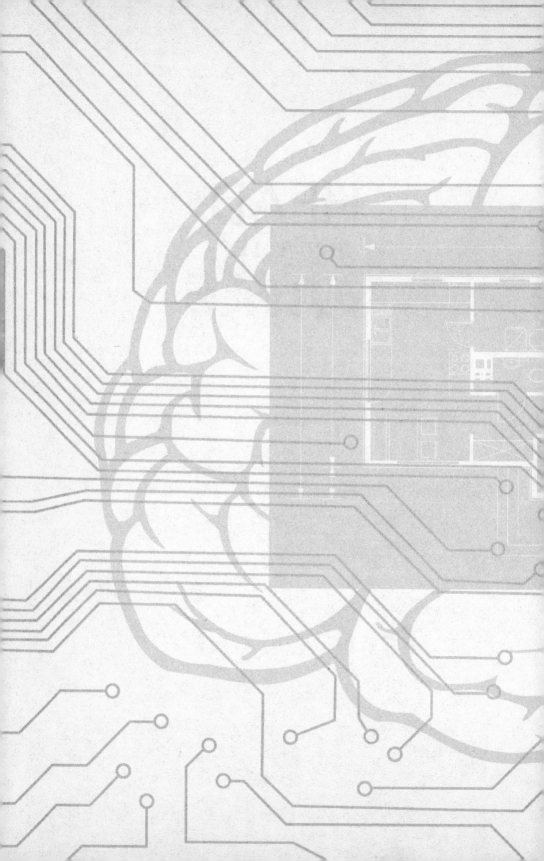

HEAD

IN THE

GAME

THE MENTAL ENGINEERING OF THE
WORLD'S GREATEST ATHLETES

BRANDON SNEED

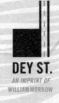

DEY ST.
AN IMPRINT OF
WILLIAM MORROW

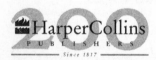

HEAD IN THE GAME. Copyright © 2017 by Brandon Sneed. All rights reserved. Printed in the United States of America. No part of this book may be used or reproduced in any manner whatsoever without written permission except in the case of brief quotations embodied in critical articles and reviews. For information address HarperCollins Publishers, 195 Broadway, New York, NY 10007.

HarperCollins books may be purchased for educational, business, or sales promotional use. For information please e-mail the Special Markets Department at SP-sales@harpercollins.com.

FIRST EDITION

Designed by Paula Russell Szafranski

Frontispiece art © takito/Shutterstock.com

Part opener art © Teamdaddy/Shutterstock.com

Library of Congress Cataloging-in-Publication Data has been applied for.

ISBN 978-0-06-245593-2

17 18 19 20 21 RS/LSC 10 9 8 7 6 5 4 3 2 1

To Katie, my wife, for always believing
and for all the other reasons you already know.

And to our kids. Some of what this book holds may
be outdated by the time you care to read it, but at the
very least, I hope this explains some things.

This is almost like a hidden world of stuff that, if you don't know about it, then you don't know anything about it. And that's really unfortunate. There's so much power we have, if we have the right tools.

—*Dr. Leslie Sherlin, cofounder and chief science officer, SenseLabs*

You have to know the world before you can act upon it.

—*Herb Yoo, cofounder and chief technical officer, Senaptec*

CONTENTS

Prologue: The Conspiracy

"'Ello, mate!"

Wearing a long, loose white T-shirt, black skinny jeans, and flip-flops, Andy Walshe, Ph.D., an enthusiastic, balding, white-haired Australian with energy for days, strolls into the Red Bull North America headquarters lobby.

I'm relieved. It's February 2016, and I was nervous that Walshe, Red Bull's director of high performance, would cancel. Not that I think Walshe is flaky—it's just that I'm here to talk with him about some things that I've tried to talk with hundreds of athletes and trainers about over the past year, and virtually none of them wanted to. These *things* sound unbelievable and have—supposedly—been helping athletes do the unthinkable, such as looking at their minds and brains and making them, in essence, more athletic. Athletes are using various machines, equipment, and software to do everything from testing their brainpower to inserting themselves into virtual worlds wherein they can train with all the mental stress and fear and challenges that they would face in the arena. Some of these things can literally look at their brains in action and sync them with their smartphones. The brain, in the palm of the hand.

These devices aren't only being used by fringe athletes looking for a gimmicky way to get ahead either: household names, from dozens of sports around the world, are using them. Tom Brady. LeBron James. Steph Curry. Kerri Walsh Jennings, the legendary Olympic beach volleyball player who calls these innovations "life-changing." Jason Day, who *has* had them change his life, becoming the number one golfer in the world in 2015 after using one. I could keep going, with examples of both men and women, in dozens of sports—football, hockey, baseball, soccer, golf, tennis, surfing, skateboarding, UFC, myriad Olympic events.

My problem, however, is that none of them have wanted to talk to me about . . . well, there are so many tools for this sort of training that they have no single clean label, so I've gone with the extremely scientific term *This Stuff.* Ever since I first stumbled across some of This Stuff a few years ago, I've been calling athletes, coaches, trainers, and so on who use it. At first, they seemed excited—and then, I don't know if they had an agent or a coach or someone else talk them out of it—but suddenly they changed their minds. Many people, "after consideration," canceled interviews. That was on top of hundreds of others who either told me no or flat-out ignored me. Stonewalled all around.

"It's a conspiracy, mate!" Walshe joked over the phone a month and a half ago.

If I was smart, I probably would have moved on, but I couldn't. For one thing, I felt like I'd stumbled into some sort of sci-fi alternate universe. For another, I wasn't just finding cool stuff that could help athletes, but stuff that could help everyone. The more I learned, the more I needed to know, because as dramatic as it feels to say this, This Stuff started to seem like it might even be important for people beyond sports, too.

That, more than anything, is why Walshe agreed to meet: This Stuff is helping athletes win championships and medals, sure, but it's also having a stunning effect on their lives. He says, "This isn't just about sports. This is about the good of humanity. I mean, we're getting into some next-level shit here."

As Walshe guides me through the Red Bull facility and we pound espressos, he *raves* about athletes reaching within themselves in unprecedented ways that often take them *beyond* themselves. Next-level shit indeed.

To get to the Red Bull performance lab and gym, we walk through a hallway. On a wall in that hallway is a massive logo: silhouetted in white against a black background, a minimalistic depiction of six stages of human evolution, from hunched-over caveman to upright human, followed by three dots, and then the next stage: a question mark.

So, the obvious question: *Why?*

"As humans, we can only train four things," Dr. Michael Gervais told me by phone one day in early 2016. Walshe put me in touch with him. Gervais—an athletic middle-aged surfer with a thick head of brown hair—is a prominent sports psychologist based in Marina del Rey. He's worked with Red Bull athletes many times, including helping "Fearless" Felix Baumgartner leap from space for Red Bull Stratos in 2012. He currently serves as the Seattle Seahawks' sports psychologist, and he works regularly with the likes of Kerri Walsh Jennings and many other elite athletes around the world.

"We can train our body, we can train our craft, we can train our spirit, and we can train our mind," Gervais says. "Until recent times, we have been remiss on very clear and very practical strategies for performers to be able to train their mind."

But how things have changed in recent times.

Until the last seventy-five years or so, you practiced a sport by, well, doing that sport. That was it. Then, over the last few decades, innovations in fitness and technology have enabled athletes to undergo ever more specific, specialized training in weight lifting, nutrition, and all manner of physical conditioning. Now athletes are constantly in the gym, in the film room, and so on, trying to snag nanoseconds' and inches' worth of advantages. And of course, that sort of training still matters and probably always will, but every possible physical advantage seems to have been mastered, exploited, and exhausted. I mean, swimmers shave their bodies to gain advantage.

On an individual level, there's always more to learn, but in general, our knowledge of how to push athletes' bodies has been maxed out. If you were to put the world's best athletes through various physical tests in a lab, in all likelihood, most would test within a few percentage points of each other. And of course, come game time, often the guys who *look* like the best athletes aren't always the best players anyway. No disrespect to the supremely conditioned Tim Tebow, but if ever hard work and competitive fire and Captain America's body added up to winning football games, Tebow would've won every Super Bowl since he got drafted in 2010.

Now, with such thin margins of physical advantage at the elite levels of sport, athletes are turning to This Stuff to get better by way of their brain, the last gap left to exploit. This is the next natural stage of athletes' evolution. They now pursue a certain mental athleticism.

To this end, This Stuff goes beyond sports into life, which, in many cases, is exactly the point. Walshe's goal, which seems to be the goal of any good performance coach, is not only to make an athlete better in his or her sport, but to make their lives better: what helps someone's life helps them perform, and what helps someone perform often helps their life.

And what is life, Walshe says, if not a performance of sorts? "Performance is all in the definition," he says. "It's performance, going after an Olympic gold medal, same as it's performance having the patience and compassion to be more present with your family and friends and children. It's the same thing."

I roughly organized all of This Stuff into four sections, according to the four ways we can train: Mind. Body. Craft. Spirit. Some of it overlaps from one category to another, which was inevitable, so I've logged my findings under each section according to how they help that particular part of a person, often by using one of the other parts. I won't be including *everything* that falls under a particular category—that would get redundant and boring. Instead, my goal is an overview that explores some of the most compelling pieces of This Stuff by way of the incredible—and sometimes literally unbelievable—stories of athletes using it with remarkable results.

As I learned all of this, I felt . . . well, I felt a lot of things. First, awe. And then—I'm not proud to admit—a brief, though very real, raging jealousy. *Where was this for ME ten years ago?!* This whole search began, in large part, because I was a pro baseball prospect myself, and a hard worker, putting on nearly fifty pounds of muscle over four years in college—only to have those dreams derailed by anxiety, depression, and obsessive-compulsive disorder. Thankfully, I'm doing much better now, but I still have moments of enormous struggle, which is a big part of what motivated me during this search.

But then I just felt foolish. Even if I didn't use This Stuff back then, how did I go so *long* thinking it was somehow worthwhile to invest so much in my body, and yet invest in nothing that helped keep my head in the game?

And then I was just confused. Why did it take so *long* for me, an athlete obsessed with figuring out the best ways to do anything, to learn about any of this?

That confusion deepened as I started calling athletes and teams to talk about it, only to be met with profound secrecy.

It's a conspiracy, mate!

Truth is, I learned, it's less conspiracy and more human nature. The tech might be new, but not the knowledge, or at least not most of it. Some is even ancient. There is a fringe subculture of people out there called "biohackers" and "neurohackers" and the like, who have been exploring some of This Stuff for some time now—but even then, it's only in the last few years that we have seen any of it trickle into sports.

A couple days before I met Walshe, I was in Portland, Oregon, to see Dr. Herb Yoo, a scientist who worked at Nike before starting Senaptec, a cutting-edge company using futuristic technology to help athletes make their brains work faster. One problem with all of this science and its application, Yoo says, is that nobody can agree on standardized ways to test and measure such things: "Even if you have some data and you want to share it with other people doing the same thing, you can't always, because you could be using different techniques, different methodologies, different types of equipment. So if Babe Ruth was evaluated with one set of tools, and somebody else—Ty Cobb, or whoever—was measured in different units, different measurements, how are you supposed to compare the two? It's just a lack of standardization. There's no agreement on how to evaluate an athlete's mind, brain, sensory performance, and etc."

Another problem seems to be that This Stuff has been around for decades, but, Yoo says, "It's been in laboratories, and people have been holding it secret, because it's their competitive advantage."

Even as "it" now makes its way out of the lab, that desire for competitive advantage is one of the biggest reasons for why I had such a hard time getting athletes to open up about using it. Where the Andy Walshes of the world see a boon for mankind, a way for humanity to move forward, many athletes, their teams, and researchers have found a secret weapon that they want to *stay* secret.

The petulant teenager in me wanted to blow that right up.

But then there's the third reason why athletes don't want to talk about This Stuff. Until recently, it has come in forms that have been so clinical and uncomfortable, and flat-out weird, that only the most die-hard *biohackers* were willing to give it a shot. Yoo's business partner Joe Bingold says, "The concepts have been around for decades. We're making [them] more accessible and convenient." And there's still a certain geeky, New Age whiff around a lot of This Stuff.

But even beyond the strangeness factor, there's a simpler reason, which is the same reason it takes guys like me forever to get help, and why so many never get any help at all: it's scary. For an athlete or coach to come out and say he is using some of This Stuff would almost certainly require him or her to acknowledge *why*—and that's more unsettling, even more terrifying, than getting naked.

When I started researching all of this a couple years ago, I did not expect it to become as time-consuming and intensive as it did.

I collected thousands of pages' worth of articles from academic and scientific journals, I collected a small library's worth of books (including more than one book from the For Dummies series), and I logged more than a thousand hours of interviews.

In the end, I focused on what applies directly to athletes, for a couple of reasons. For one, I want to see how the big world of sports is rapidly changing, and for the better, and how, one way or another, what helps athletes ends up helping all of us. For all the *biohacking* and whatnot going on out there, athletes, like most of us, don't have time to waste on research, methods, or tools that don't seem to have a direct and relatively immediate impact on their performance.

Even so, I had my brain hooked to a computer, and on a few separate occasions, electrocuted. I had needles shoved into my scalp. I spent thousands of dollars running around North America and testing dozens of options as I tried to answer questions that might not even have answers. Sometimes I felt like an addict consumed only by the thought of my next fix. I spent hours in sensory deprivation chambers, in which, more than once, I may have lost my mind.

What I'm saying is, consider yourself warned.

What I've found, however, is a dazzling look at the future, the crux of it boiling down to something that Herb Yoo said to me: "You have to know the world before you can act upon it."

Because look, and here's the guts of the whole matter: This Stuff shows us that for athletes—and so for anyone—"getting their mind right" or "getting their head in the game" (or whatever other cliché you prefer) isn't a nebulous concept, separate from the physical part of a person. This Stuff throws into sharp focus exactly how the mental aspects of a human being are every bit as real as, say, their muscles. The mind flows through the brain like air through the lungs, like blood through the heart. And This Stuff shows people the world within their heads, that they may act upon it.

Much of this left me in awe of how much power it seems athletes may actually have to make themselves better. Sometimes I was also left in an almost tearful rage at people who have been hiding the details of this new frontier.

But mostly, it left me giddy with wonder and hope for what's coming next, and not only in sports, but also for myself—which is to say, for all of us.

PART ONE

THE MIND

Chapter 1

Two Very Different Brains

It's the 2015 NFC Championship game, and Seattle Seahawks quarterback Russell Wilson lines up in shotgun with a nearly impossible task ahead. The Seahawks, the defending Super Bowl champions, have just gotten the ball back from the Green Bay Packers at the thirty-one-yard line, and they are losing 19–7 with only one time-out and 3:52 left to play.

That's a lot to think about. A lot of pressure on young shoulders.

So far in his short career, Wilson's shown he can handle it. After all, he was the Seahawks' starting quarterback last year in only his second season as a pro, and he's one of the less likely rising stars in the league, proving a lot of people wrong with every game he and the Hawks win. He's physically talented, with above-average arm strength and accuracy, and he moves well, but even so, he's been doubted for some time now, even losing his job as a starting quarterback in *college* a few short years ago. He was a middling draft pick in 2012, selected in the third round seemingly as an afterthought behind several other much-hyped quarterback prospects. Most people thought that his talent wasn't enough to make up for one glaring and uncontrollable weakness: he's short for the NFL, less than six feet tall in a league where the average quarterback is six-three. Analysts and pundits called him a waste of a pick. ESPN graded the Hawks' choice a C-, CBS Sports a D, Bleacher Report an F.

And tonight, Wilson has lived down to expectations, throwing for a paltry seventy-five yards, running for an even more paltry five, getting sacked four times, throwing zero touchdowns—and throwing a nightmare *four* interceptions.

So if ever there is a time to turn things around, it's now.

After running back Marshawn Lynch runs for fourteen yards, Wilson and the rest of the Hawks hustle into position, in an urgent no-huddle offense now. Next play, Wilson throws to wide receiver Doug Baldwin for twenty yards. Play after that, incompletion. Then Lynch beats his man down the sideline, and Wilson throws a gorgeous thirty-five-yard lob that lands soft in Lynch's hands. Lynch jukes a tackler and drags another into the end zone. TOUCHDOWN.

But then replay shows that Lynch stepped out of bounds at the nine.

Lynch runs for four yards, then, unshaken, Wilson runs into the end zone to score. There's 2:09 left on the clock.

Then the Seahawks convert an onside kick.

Wilson runs for seventeen yards, Lynch runs for another three, Wilson throws for eight more, and then he hands off to Lynch, who runs the last twenty-four yards for another touchdown.

Suddenly, with 1:25 left in the game, the Hawks have gone from desperate and running out of time to in the lead with too much time.

Up 20–19, they can't count on Aaron Rodgers and the Packers to not at *least* make it into field goal range, so instead of kicking the extra point, they're going for two.

In shotgun, Wilson takes the snap and rolls right, scanning the field, searching for an open receiver, but there's already a Packer defender in his face. The play has totally fallen apart. Wilson's got nowhere to go by air or by land, and he's about to be sacked. For him to panic right now and just drop to the ground to soften the blow would be perfectly acceptable.

But he doesn't. He ducks and spins left.

The defender stays on him in hot pursuit, and there's another right behind him.

Wilson turns again, now running almost directly *backward*. He hits the fifteen-yard line, thirteen yards from where the play began. Another half turn and he's back at the seventeen-yard line, still dancing away. "In big trouble," deadpans Fox television announcer Joe Buck.

Another defender flies in and latches his arms around Wilson's legs, and as he starts to fall he slings the ball across the field. Buck says how it looks for everyone watching: *"Just up for grabs!"*

But it isn't. In the chaos, Wilson has somehow seen tight end Luke Willson on the far side of the field, guarded but open enough to score if he gets a good enough pass. Russell gives it to him. Willson fights off a defender, catches the pass at the one-yard line, and turns into the end zone.

Everyone goes nuts. It's an all-time great, ridiculous, clutch play.

The Packers kick a field goal before time expires, and the game goes into overtime, where the first score wins.

The Hawks get the ball first, but the Packers' kickoff coverage is strong and pins them deep, at the thirteen-yard line. Lynch runs for four yards, then Wilson throws to Doug Baldwin for ten yards, which Lynch follows with another four-yard run. And then Wilson gets sacked, sending them to third down. Fail to convert, and they probably have to punt to the Packers.

Wilson throws a thirty-five-yard bomb, again to Baldwin.

The next play, another bomb, also for thirty-five yards—and the game-winning touchdown.

For those last few minutes, Wilson was perfect, drawing on deep reserves of preternatural calm and ruthless efficiency that have since become known as his hallmarks. His teammates like to say that he's probably half robot, and some of them sound like they're only half joking.

Of all his strengths, this might be Wilson's most important: he is stunningly good at ruling his emotions instead of letting them rule him. When he was a late draft pick selected by a team that had recently spent a lot of money on another free agent QB, and when he was scorned for that, and when he became successful and people said he really wasn't that important to the Seahawks as they won the Super Bowl the year before, and when he threw all those interceptions against the Packers, he never got emotional. Maybe the most emotional he's been since he was drafted was after that comeback, when he wept.

During that comeback, and particularly that incredible two-point conversion, Wilson faced enormous pressure, and things spun out of control in a critical moment of a game during which he had struggled greatly—and yet he never lost control of himself. He and his brain and his body were all in perfect sync, each helping the other, all of them working together. That scene is the epitome of good performance, and it's a perfect metaphor for this book. How did Wilson face that crushing adversity and still do . . . *that*?

That's beyond mastering a game. That is mastering the mind.

In the fall of 2014, a few months after I started researching any of this, I came across an old *ESPN The Magazine* article that gave me my first real handle on this mountain of mind-brain information. It was a profile of the Seattle Seahawks. The headline:

"Lotus Pose on Two." The lead photo: Wilson doing yoga in full uniform.

The story was about head coach Pete Carroll's overarching philosophy of "a happy player is a better player," geared around Wilson and the Hawks using meditation, visualization, and yoga, their weekly meetings with a psychologist, how they cut practices short so players can get more sleep, how they play weird "brain training" iPad games, and featured wide receiver Doug Baldwin throwing around words like *prefrontal cortex*.

The writer described it all as "a bizarro football world."

The general consensus seemed to be that it was all some kind of hippielike way of trying to do football differently. Nobody expected much out of the Hawks that year either, remember, or for Wilson to matter much as an NFL quarterback. So it's not all that surprising that the writer, and then the general public's reaction after the article ran, didn't know quite what to make of all of that, which sounded like more or less snake-oil-y psychobabble. And then, of course, that very season, Carroll and Wilson—with plenty of heavy lifting from running back Marshawn Lynch and their defense—went on to win the Super Bowl.

People that article mentioned later told me that the writer missed much of what the Hawks were really doing. Yoga, meditation, meticulously plotted sleep schedules, working knowledge of prefontal cortices, Carroll saying things like "quiet your mind"—all of those things were merely visible manifestations of deeper science at work, waves on the surface of an ocean of research teeming with answers to the very questions I was asking—and far more answers than I would have even dared to hope were out there.

And that was only the beginning.

Every new thread of a story seemed to tug at a whole new ball of yarn, to the tune of hundreds if not thousands of athletes in dozens of sports the world over. I found one story after another of men and women using one piece or another of This Stuff, some of these athletes already legends and trying to get even better, and others who were comparatively average, downright underdogs, who have then defeated the legends to become legends themselves.

At some point, I became so inundated with such stories that I no longer saw This Stuff as a novel *enhancement* to what athletes were already doing, but rather as a necessity other athletes were missing. Or, to put it another way, the idea of training the body without also directly training the mind began to seem like choosing a half measure.

At this point, This Stuff no longer seemed like a possible trend destined to flame out in a few years. It seemed like a revolution: I felt like I had, completely by accident, stumbled across a new frontier in performance enhancement. "This is almost like a hidden world of stuff that, if you don't know about it, then you don't know anything about it," says Dr. Leslie Sherlin, the CEO and CSO of SenseLabs, a company that has worked with Red Bull and creates technology that gives athletes a way to look at their brains by using their iPhone. "And that's really unfortunate. There's so much power we have, if we have the right tools."

That power, as these tools show, undoes one of the long-standing, most frightening elements of facing one's mental needs: that unlike, say, an ankle sprain, confronting a psychological challenge feels like confronting something within yourself that might not only be damaged, but unfixable. If you're broken but can't be fixed, would you really want to know? (And, for that matter, would you want anyone else to know?)

Until recently, even the world's leading scientists believed that whatever state someone's brain was in, that's the state in which it would remain until the end of their days.

But that all changed about fifteen years ago, with a revolution in neuroscience.

About two decades ago—which is virtually last week in the world of science—scientists knew, without a doubt, that by the time we reached our twenties, our brains—and thus our minds, our personalities—were set, unchangeable, for better or worse. *It's just how we're wired,* was the conventional wisdom.

In the mid-1980s, however, the foundation for that belief was already beginning to crumble, thanks to neuroscientist Dr. Michael Merzenich. While studying how monkeys adapt to injuries, Merzenich saw the physical landscape of their brains change.

That was supposed to be impossible.

So impossible, in fact, that when Merzenich announced what he'd found, his fellow scientists reacted by, more or less, mocking him and labeling him, at best, a dummy, and at worst a liar.

Well, Merzenich possessed unique drive and passion and, apparently, a real rebel streak that rivals anyone in sports (or anyone, period). He raged against the establishment, spending the next twenty *years* working to prove his theory to the world until, finally, his fellow scientists said he was right.

Now, they call it "neuroplasticity." It's almost like Merzenich was sent back in time to change our future. That's how big his discovery was. If our brain itself can experience literal, physical change—if the physical layout and function of the brain can be reengineered—then that means Who We Are can change, too. We are no longer at the mercy of our brain. All of our worst moments can, more or less, be traced to some wiring gone awry in our heads—and neuroplasticity means we can change that wiring. Our brains don't have to control us. We can control them.

That concept is the cornerstone of all This Stuff. Athletes don't have to just hope they *get in the zone* or *go unconscious* or, to go with the latest hip "peak performance" jargon, *get into "flow."*

Hungarian psychologist Mihaly Csikszentmihalyi ("Me-high Chick-sent-me-high") coined the term in his 1990 book *Flow,* calling it "the secret to happiness." Journalist Steven Kotler expanded on that with his 2014 book, *The Rise of Superman,* in which he insists that flow is *the* key to success in life.

Now, though, I'm not so certain that chasing flow is as productive as building a better brain. Using This Stuff, athletes can train to do just that, meaning they can be great even *without* flow—and more easily slip into it when they really need it.

To put it frankly, the more you learn about This Stuff, the more it starts to feel like a gift beamed down by God, saying, "Here's a little help everyone, enjoy!"

However, before any of this can make anyone better, they have to first make sure their brain is healthy. When your brain works *against* you instead of with you, you can become convinced that struggling at a game is a matter of life or death. That starts to feel like hell, and that's nothing compared to what your brain does to your life outside the game, shading the way you see the world like it's gone through some sort of murky and discolored Photoshop.

I know how badly your mind can break you because mine broke me.

This is not a story I wanted to put into print, but leaving it out would feel dishonest. When my hunt for This Stuff began about three years ago, it was personal, and many people only opened up after they heard some of my story. It seemed to unlock an unspoken trust. *If this guy's digging up other athletes' secrets, at least he's willing to trade some of his own.*

Like a billion other kids, I grew up dreaming about being a big-league ballplayer. The oldest of five children, I grew up in a classic small Southern town in eastern North Carolina. My parents were devout Christians, holding weekly Bible studies attended by hundreds of people, starting a church, and hosting large Christian conventions. I was raised accordingly. Among many things I was taught was that God gives favor to those who honor Him. An earnest child eager to please, to put it mildly, I honored the heck out of Him.

Sometimes it really felt like I had that favor. I played varsity high school baseball starting in eighth grade, and varsity basketball and soccer from freshman year on, and my favorite days were the ones when the games came easy: when baseballs looked like beach balls, when basketball rims felt like ball pits, when I felt a gear faster than the rest of the world around me and my body was not my body but an instrument at my command. When I played my best, I felt free, and walk-off home runs and state championships and all other manner of great things happened.

I was a good enough baseball player to regularly make summer league all-star, travel, and showcase teams. I was better than most guys on the field any given day, but I wasn't a superstar, and some days I struggled, and when I struggled I struggled hard, and it compounded upon itself, a million mental layers wide.

To get better, instead of playing soccer and basketball my senior year, I spent that time working out at Triple Crown, a local indoor baseball facility in a big warehouse with a turf infield, a few bullpens, a few batting cages, a weight room, all that. My American Legion coach, Mullis, ran the place. One day in early spring, after I'd been throwing and hitting and all that with my best friend, also named Brandon, Mullis called me to the front desk to introduce me to a college scout. The scout was in his fifties or so, with gray hair, a ball cap, and wearing khakis and a polo shirt, looking like your classic old-school, wizened baseball scout. I don't remember our conversation exactly, but from what I do remember, he shook my hand and studied it, then asked if my other hand was just as big. I didn't realize he was joking until after I'd pulled my left hand out of my catcher's mitt and held it up to his face.

The scout laughed and said nice things about the size of my forearms and my strong arm and quick bat and raw power and blah blah blah, and he asked me how tall I was and how much I weighed. I told him a little lie, saying I was six-foot-one—which was true, when I was wearing cleats anyway—and that I weighed 175, when really I was only around 165. The scout said if I worked with a good college coach, and polished my game, and got in the gym and put on some muscle, and had a good season, he'd probably sign me. And he said he knew just the coach, a former professional catcher and outfielder at a small Division II college up the road.

The scout called Coach right then and there. Coach said if the scout liked me, I was worth a workout; a week or two later, Coach said he wanted me to play for him. He told me he had no scholarship money left and that I'd be competing against three other incoming freshmen for the starting job. He added, though, that he'd be surprised if I didn't win the starting spot, and if I did well, I'd get a scholarship the next year—and the scout said not to let all that bother me anyway, because pro teams often pay off college debt for their prospects anyway. That was good enough for me.

A couple of months later, my high school team won the state championship, and the star player on the team we beat was going to be one of my main competitors for playing time in college, which I took as a good sign.

That summer, however, I didn't play well for my American Legion team, and my main competition for playing time was a catcher going to a big Division I school on a scholarship—and then when he got hurt, my coach, Mullis, still benched me for a younger catcher. I was struggling that bad. Those old feelings of having to prove myself welled back up, irrational and relentless as ever.

It hurt, but we went on to win the American Legion state championship. Later, Mullis took me to Chick-Fil-A and we talked about it. He knew I wasn't happy about not getting to play as much—after all, he had convinced me to play for him after watching me go through a terrible experience for another American Legion team the summer before, getting treated poorly by coaches and players alike. He said I had as much raw power and talent as anyone, but for reasons he couldn't figure out, I seemed scared of it.

That would continue in kind in college.

Everything started off well enough. I worked hard, which Coach liked, and he told me I looked like an All-American. I got obsessed with every aspect—or what I thought was every aspect—of being a great baseball player. I became an expert in fitness, in hitting, in everything. I spent hours working out every day. During my freshman year, I put on 20 pounds, and by my senior year, 35 more, going from 165 pounds to 220 while making sure what I put on was good weight, too, meticulously monitoring my body fat, which stayed around 6 to 8 percent. My teammates thought I was using HGH or steroids. The scout saw me at Pro Days and tryouts, and said he liked what he saw more every year—but he needed me to have that good season.

Problem was, I wasn't even having average seasons. I went from maybe-an-All-American to, for a few truly awful weeks, not even making the travel squad. When I was good, I was clearly the best catcher on the team, but I was so erratic, and the other catchers were consistent. Although I was bitter about it for some time, I can't blame Coach for playing them over me.

I don't remember how the downturn happened, exactly, or why. I do remember a bad intersquad scrimmage, and then a bad practice, and then all of a sudden it was snowballing and I couldn't make it stop. I'd gotten that same feeling from high school, feeling like I had to play great or I wouldn't play at all, only now it seemed even worse. I tried too hard again. All my old insecurities flooded back up. I could not stop overthinking everything, and not just in baseball. I struggled at life itself, the bulk of which revolved the cliché doubts of a naive Christian college kid's eyes opening up and he begins questioning his religious upbringing and all that it demands of him. My emotions over this were likely compounded by my sensitive nature, not to mention my parents' only advice at the time being, more or less, "keep believing" and "just have faith."

And here's where we come to the flip side of the story, when everything feels cursed against you, when your body is not your body but some kind of enemy, when nothing is easy, when the laws of the universe feel rewritten to conspire against you.

My fears, both on and off the field, grew worse and worse until they physically manifested themselves by way of the Yips. You ever seen the movie *Major League II*? We watched it on the bus every road trip. There's this character, a catcher named Rube Baker, who can't throw the ball back to the pitcher. The Yips, they call it. Same as guys who can't make a putt or hit a free throw or kick a field goal, Rube had a nightmare case of the Yips.

One of my nicknames was "Rube."

I always had a cannon of an arm—one of my best traits; I loved picking runners off second who took too large of leads, sometimes from my knees—but ever since Little League, for some reason, that toss back to the mound always made me nervous, and it started getting worse in high school. One rainy afternoon during an American Legion game the summer before my senior year, a throw to the pitcher got away from me, and the pitcher gave me hell. Then it kept happening, and before long, every throw came with a minor panic attack that made me so tense I felt like my throwing shoulder got stuck.

Through my freshman year of college, my brain felt like some sort of steadily burning fire. I came to imagine little dragons flying around in my skull, going nuts. I felt lost and helpless. Coach didn't know how to help. My parents tried, but they didn't know how to help. Books I read didn't help. The Bible didn't help. Church didn't help. God didn't help. People back home were just confused when they saw how much I was struggling, and they didn't know how to help.

I felt like I had Yips with everything. I screwed up signals, blew easy plays, sailed throws into the outfield. Sometimes I felt like I'd forgotten how to swing a bat. One time—I'm not making this up—when I was on first base, desperate to do something good, I tagged up on a pop fly to the catcher. Even off the field, I became a head case. I felt like I didn't even know how to just . . . hang out. Just be a dude. Pickup basketball, something I once loved, made me so tense I could barely function. Some days, just driving, I'd be squeezing the steering wheel as tight as I could without realizing it until my hand began to cramp.

I never had a good season.

There were a few good games with a few good plays, some runners thrown out, some home runs hit—one game I even hit for the cycle—and a few times I snuck my way into the heart of the lineup. But eventually Coach, a good but old-school man, basically shrugged and said, *"I guess you just don't have the mind for this."* I don't remember my statistics, but I'm pretty sure I never hit better than .200, never hit more than a couple home runs a season, and certainly never was an All-American.

After I graduated in May 2009, I still should have been happy. Life was good. I married my longtime good friend Katie. She was gorgeous and smart and a heck of an athlete herself (varsity basketball and softball team captain three years running, All-State in both, Wendy's High School Heisman nominee, could've played either sport in college just about anywhere if she'd wanted to). We'd met when we were ten after my family moved down the street from hers, into a house her father built. I'd been in love with her basically ever since, but we didn't date until the summer between our sophomore and junior years of college, by which point she was down in Georgia, going to the Savannah College of Art and Design, and we were living six hours apart during the school year. We'd started hanging out a lot again that summer, and then one day, when I was about to leave her house, she stole my keys so that I couldn't go. I chased her until we ended up by her parents' pool, where I grabbed her and we almost fell in, and then we kissed.

I was happy at times, but so often, and seemingly more often every passing month, my little mind dragons kept starting their fires. Part of why I fell in love with Katie was that I felt like myself with her—goofy, happy, carefree—which was ever more rare. With her I was at peace. But as time went by, that faded, too, the dragon fire burning ever hotter.

What has haunted me wasn't that I failed. Failure, if nothing else, makes for good stories.

What haunted me was *why* I had failed.

I felt like there were two of me, with the "real," good Brandon getting pushed around by this other guy who was insecure, and afraid to reckon with himself, and who compensated by acting arrogant and bullylike so as not to reveal his true nature. I didn't just get nervous or have a flash of temper, like all of us—it was like, when that other guy showed up, he took over. The longer Katie and I were married, the more like a jerk I behaved. I'd walk around with this swagger, shoulders thrown back, chest puffed out, talking all about me, never asking about her. In retrospect, my problem was obvious: that was all a shield.

Inside, I was a coward.

I tried distracting myself for a while. Work. Church. Coaching. Charity work. Things I loved as a kid, when I was a goofball who just did things to make people smile. But they didn't make me happy anymore.

I couldn't let baseball go, even though I wanted to. When I was alone and things were quiet, I kept thinking about how much I had worked and sacrificed, and how it all felt for nothing. Every bad play in pickup basketball and every error in rec league softball, every punk talking trash and trying to cheat—they all set my head on fire again. I'd daydream about car accidents that left me paralyzed so I no longer had the option of wishing I could play.

I knew the way I was thinking wasn't normal and that I probably needed professional help, but that was scary, too, and only got my mind dragons more agitated.

So I distracted myself more, steadily becoming less noble and more cliché. I didn't even know *why* I was doing what I was doing half the time.

I doubt anyone other than Katie noticed. I was good at covering up. People might have seen the occasional temper during softball or basketball—but at home, there was lying, and yelling, and pain, and tears, and regret, to the point where Katie said she was having a hard time recognizing me. When your wife doesn't recognize you, you need help. But I still didn't get it on my own. Katie had to finally say *enough.* If I wanted us to survive, I had to get help. It wasn't an ultimatum, it was a fact. She was going to lose me, because I was already losing myself.

We went to one of the most frightening places in the world.

Therapy.

It took time. It was painful. Mind surgery, no anesthetic, picking apart the hollow shell of a man I was pretending to be. But then we could see where the broken parts were, and how they happened, and what could be done about them.

In time, it worked. First and foremost, it *gave answers*. Depression. Anxiety. Obsessive-compulsive disorder. Maybe more.

I saw my mind monsters' seeds, their roots, the ways they grew up in me. I saw, at the root of it all, a psychological black hole of fear. And I learned. I saw where the monsters were born and what helped them grow. I did something I once thought inconceivable, agreeing to prescription medication—and it immediately helped. Finding the right mix took time—Celexa, then Zoloft, now Buspar and Luvox—and I weathered some undesirable and embarrassing side effects. But it was worth it.

I still have moments, and I can be exhausting, and neurotic, and needy, and moody, and I've had to ask for more than my fair share of forgiveness. However, I believe that Katie making me go to therapy not only saved our marriage—she might have also saved my life.

Then, a couple years after I began therapy, in October 2013, Katie became pregnant. And, as I imagine happens with most men who first learn they are fathers, the current version of myself suddenly felt hugely lacking.

Taking medication and talking through problems had been useful, but the more Katie's belly grew, the less adequate my treatment felt. My therapist told me that I was "breaking generational curses." I'd heard that saying in church, but she showed me science: our parents' struggles, and their parents' before them, by way of our DNA, also become our own.

Even if my genes didn't pass my problems on, however, I felt a need to know more, and to be stronger. I imagined future conversations with my son if he started to struggle. *Well, son, I have this problem, and you might, too, but we can deal with it.*

How, Daddy?

I could not imagine having nothing more to say than, *Well, you can talk to someone who knows a lot about it, and you might have to take pills all your life, and have faith.*

Something about that felt dishonest.

I became convinced that what people had told me so far was, if not *wrong*, then at least incomplete. Surely, we are capable of doing more for the mind than merely accepting what we have. I don't know where this certainty came from. Maybe I'm just stubborn. All I know for sure is that Coach's old criticism kept echoing in my head—*you don't have the mind for this*—and I felt like arguing. Maybe I didn't have the mind for it *yet*, but couldn't I have trained it up somehow? Surely, I thought, there had to be *something* we could do for ourselves.

At the very least—if all we could do was throw our hands up and "give it all to God"—I needed to find the limits of what we *could* do. After all, I reasoned, I learned how to build my body. Why could I not do the same for my mind?

I started thinking a lot about great athletes—not so that I could recapture a shattered dream, or make my son able to do what I failed to do, or anything so delusional. I'd made my peace with baseball. I don't regret failing at it. I regret forgetting to have fun, and I regret making life harder than it should have been for people I loved. But I wasn't hung up on the game. Rather, baseball, and sports on the whole, became a metaphor for all my hopes and dreams.

So I needed to know: What is it in great athletes—in all of us—that makes a mind strong? And how can the mind be made stronger?

I had no idea there were actually so many answers.

Chapter 2

A Way Beyond the Labels

One afternoon in mid-December 2015, I leave home in Greenville, North Carolina, and drive an hour and a half west to the office of Dr. Dan Chartier, a psychologist in Raleigh.

I'm here for something that I first learned the Seattle Seahawks were doing with SenseLabs and Dr. Michael Gervais: EEG assessment and training. These are not simple procedures.

Chartier follows a bleary-eyed woman out into the lobby, wishes her well, then welcomes me with a big smile and walks me back down a hallway to his office. He's a slim man, of average height, bald, with a neatly trimmed white beard. His voice is deep and calm and confident, and he laughs easily.

I sit in a leather chair, he sits in a swivel chair at a computer desk, and a few minutes of chitchat later, Chartier straps a blue skullcap to my head. There's a long set of wires attached to the cap; they connect to a computer on the desk beside me. "This cap technology," he says, "was developed primarily for NASA, in the early days of space exploration, when humans were being put into space. The scientists involved wanted to track what was happening in their brains."

Now it's being used the same way, only instead of helping humans go into outer space, it's helping us explore the mind, that other infinite, mystifying universe.

When the cap is all set, Chartier picks up a big needle. "Now, I know you're an athlete," he says, "and you've been taught to push through the pain and whatnot, but I'm serious. If at any point during this process, you feel too much pain, *puh-leeze,* let me know. Now we're going to start with the left side of your forehead."

He sticks the needle through a sensor and into my skin, and swirls it around. This, he explains, is to "abrade" the skin—that's a nice way of saying he needs to scratch it up so the gel in the sensors actually connects with my scalp. Feels like a bugbite.

"You know," I say, "I'm starting to see why this hasn't exactly gone mainstream."

He gives me nineteen such abrasions, one per sensor.

After testing the sensor connections, Chartier turns to the computer and asks me some questions. *Are you on any medication?* Yes, I tell him—one hundred milligrams Luvox, twenty milligrams Buspar, twice daily—but as per his instructions, I haven't taken either for twenty-four hours so as not to interfere too much with his test. *Have you suffered any particularly nasty blows to the head during your life?* Nothing major, I tell him, but he expresses concern at two incidents. First, a snowboarding accident I had a couple months earlier, and years earlier while chasing down a pop fly foul ball, diving for it—and sending my forehead full speed into a railing running around the stadium.

"Well," he says, "the inside of the skull is, technically, not a very healthy place for the brain to be. Especially the frontal area. There are some protrusions there that whiplash can bounce the brain off of, and cause bruising . . . Virtually everyone has had some measure of brain trauma, from trips and falls, slips on the ice, sports, certainly car crashes, and so on. It's a wonder we survive. But this will be an objective look at what your brain is or is not doing."

Chartier double-checks all the sensors, opens a computer program, and we begin.

For about thirty minutes, working in five-minute intervals, he records my brain activity as I perform various tasks: sitting there with my eyes open, then with my eyes closed, then meditating, then reading a convoluted passage written in Old English, and doing math. The idea is to see how my brain handles simple situations, some of which are demanding and some of which are not, in order to see, generally, how it is functioning. If it's too worked up just doing *this,* for instance, then it's probably *way* too worked up during actual stress.

When we finish, Chartier pulls off the cap, cleans the sensor goop off my head, and says, "Okay, now you'll be able to officially tell people you had your head examined."

The full, technical term for this is *quantitative electroencephalography,* though "EEG" for short is fine. Our brains have about ninety billion neurons, which are brain cells that send signals to each other that are first sparked by bursts of electricity. EEG sees and records that electrical activity. You know how, in the hospital, they have that heart monitor that shows the waves of your heartbeat? EEG is similar, showing the waves of your brain. Generally, these brain waves are categorized thusly, organized according to ranges of Hertz (or cycles per second):

- 0.5–2 Hz: delta, most prominent during deep, dreamless sleep.
- 3–7 Hz: theta, most prominent in that dreamy state of half sleep, though they also sometimes ramp up during a creative rhythm.

- 8–12 Hz: alpha, most essential for athletes and other performers, dominant during calm, relaxed focus. They are super prominent when an athlete is in a flow state (or in the zone, or on automatic—whatever term you like).
- 13–40 Hz: beta, dominant during concentrated thought, rising the harder we think. Good for math or solving complex problems; bad—crippling—during a game.
- 40–100 Hz: gamma, dominant only in fleeting, über-rare moments of inspiration, joy, success, etc. Think epiphanies, or championship, gold-medal performances.

Which brain waves dominate what parts of your brain is a good indication of what's working right, and what could be better. Generally speaking, most of those ranges are present at any given time, and they seem to be a key to everything from peak performance to curing mental illnesses.

It will take Chartier some time to review all of my data, and he's pretty in demand, so I won't be able to see my full results for a month. He says he can offer me a quick preview, though. To give me my results, first, he'll look at my raw data, which first appears on-screen as a series of jagged lines, like a half-dozen different heart monitors all at once. Inevitably, there will be a few massive spikes, called "artifact," caused not by my brain's electricity but rather by the muscles in my face or head. (Stillness is key during the tests.) He'll comb through, deleting these, then plug the cleaned data into a software program, which will translate the readings into "maps" that look like my head, viewed from above.

If the brain waves fall into a "healthy" range—based off a database of hundreds of thousands of brain maps taken of "healthy" brains—then there's no color. The map is clear.

Regions less active than a healthy brain—the clinical term being *hypoactive*—appear as shades of blue. Hyperactive, shades of red.

First, for an example, Chartier opens the file of "Jim," an anonymous former client. Jim was charged with murder. His attorney brought him to Chartier because Jim had uncontrollable rage problems, and he felt that Chartier's test could shed light on why.

On his Acer computer monitor, Chartier pulls up nine different brain maps: delta, theta, alpha, SMR (sensorimotor rhythm), beta1, beta2, beta3, gamma1, and gamma2. (These are simply more detailed breakdowns of the aforementioned ranges.)

Jim's brain maps are almost all covered by shades of blue. The darker the shade, the worse off Jim is, and some of the maps look like vibrant blue planets. Poor Jim's brain is *"wayyyy* underfunctioning," Chartier says, sounding sad for him. "What that shows is, his brain doesn't gear up to do much of what a brain should be doing."

If Jim's brain was healthy, the maps would be clear. No matter how angry someone gets, a healthy brain stops them from, say, picking up the gun and getting in the car and driving to someone's house because he sold him some bad drugs. A healthy brain finds other ways to deal with the problem. "But a person whose brain looks like this, they don't think that way," Chartier says. "They don't even have the neurological underpinnings to even *think* about thinking that way."

The inverse, Chartier says, is, "People who, instead of blues, they could have bright reds and pinks, meaning that areas of the brain are overfunctioning."

"Wait," I say. "That changes how we look at why people do things they do, right?"

Chartier smiles. "Exactly. I see these horrible-looking [brain maps], pointing directly to poor inhibition, poor decision making, lacking empathy, difficulty in reading other people's feelings—

and, therefore, not appreciating when they're doing something that's causing harm. The vehement opposition the prosecution has to that kind of information is—*we just want to say he was wrong and we're gonna kill him!* Rather than, *Damn. No wonder he did what he did.* This is objective. It's science. And some people don't like science."

Jim is an extreme example, of course, but this casts a new light on all of us. When we feel out of control, maybe we really are. Maybe when we do regrettable things that we can't stop even as we're doing them, it doesn't necessarily mean we're bad people. This doesn't absolve us of wrongdoing—if anything, it gives us more responsibility to change—but it also evokes more compassion for those who do terrible things. Sure, people *can* just be "bad"—thoughts and beliefs can, and will, dictate brain function, and as Chartier says, the first step in any psychological evolution requires the patient wanting to change. But often, bad brains drive people to do things they don't even *want* to do, or prevent them from doing things they *do* want to do.

After showing me Jim's blue maps, Chartier takes a quick look at some of my data. He opens one of my files, combs through the readings quickly to remove obvious artifact, generates my maps— and then blurts, "Oh!"

There is a *whole* lot of red.

And Chartier is clearly surprised. Maybe even nervous. "That's . . . interesting!" he says. He laughs and clears his throat. "Sorry." He resumes a more clinical tone. "It's probably nothing. Really, nothing. I don't—please, don't worry about it. Yet. We'll talk about it when we meet again."

I laugh, too. *Okay, I won't, don't* you *worry about* me *worrying.* Then, being super unworried, I jabber on, asking what this *could* mean in terms of my anxiety and depression and OCD, and could it mean I maybe have *this* condition or *that* one, or maybe

I—and then Chartier stops me so that he can say something beautiful: "I hope you don't find it flippant when I say this, but I don't care so much about the diagnostic label. That's what's amazing about this stuff. It takes us beyond labels."

Labels can be useful. They can help us better comprehend things that might be otherwise incomprehensible. When someone can't breathe and they don't know why, a doctor telling them they have asthma and prescribing an inhaler can be life changing, even lifesaving. But when it comes to the mind, labels can also make us forget that it's just shaped by the brain, same as our air is filtered by our lungs. And our brain is just another organ, and sometimes one piece or another of it might need some improvement.

That's the beauty of EEG. Showing you your brain is a powerful thing in and of itself, but EEG doesn't stop there. With EEG, it is possible to take the parts of the brain that are either too weak or too active, and reengineer them to be what they need to be.

Dan Chartier has been using EEG training since the 1980s, back when it was even more fringe than it is now. He is good friends with Dr. Barry Sterman, one of the pioneers in the field. Chartier once helped a cyclist who'd been smashed by a truck overcome PTSD and get back on the road—and then she set state records. He has also seen a schizophrenic woman with fourteen different personalities coalesce into a single person. "In a way, it is a surprise," he says. "Because it's always, 'Let's hope we arrive.' But then we arrive and hey, great, we're here. It's trust in the process."

Take, for instance, all that red in my maps. If it ends up indicating that, say, my brain is generating too strong beta waves in a certain location, then Chartier can take a sensor and attach it to my scalp over that location, and then, using various computer software programs, I can train that part of my brain to calm down until it reaches a healthy level of activity.

EEG training, in other words, can take those parts shaded by reds or blues and make them clear again.

Human EEG was discovered by a German scientist named Hans Berger. Before he was a scientist, he joined the military and had a near-death experience when he was thrown from his horse into the path of a large horse-drawn artillery gun, which stopped with its wagon wheel just short of crushing him. He survived with nothing more than a terrible scare—but that night, his father sent him a telegram. His father never sent him telegrams. The telegram said that Berger's sister had been struck with sudden fear that Berger was badly hurt. Berger believed that he'd had some kind of telepathic experience with his sister. Inspired by that, he studied neuroscience, and along the way, in 1924, he produced the first recorded human brain wave in history. However, Berger was such an anxious man that he put off publishing anything about his work for five more years—and when he finally did publish, his peers in the scientific community mocked him. While battling a crippling, chronic depression, Berger kept working until he committed suicide in 1941. Tragically, it was within that decade that his work began gaining serious respect, and nowadays, as Dr. David Millett, now the program director of epilepsy at the Hoag Epilepsy Treatment Center, wrote in 2002, Berger's work ranks among "the most surprising, remarkable, and momentous developments in the history of clinical neurology."

So why, then, is EEG not a more mainstream tool? Everyone knows about pills, but start telling people about EEG training and their eyes go wide.

Part of the problem is that what I've been calling "EEG assessment" and "EEG training" goes by other names loaded with baggage, in particular the hippie-dippie type: "biofeedback" and "neurofeedback." Around the 1960s and 1970s, neurofeedback got a bad rap, in no small part because of well-meaning but zeal-ously proselytizing celebrity endorsers, such as John Lennon and Yoko Ono, who went on live television, strapped themselves into EEG equipment, and gave an "alpha training" demonstra-tion. Practitioners have recently started using other terms such as *training the brain's physiology* and the like.

I first learned much of this from *A Symphony in the Brain,* a book by science journalist Jim Robbins. Published in July 2000, followed by an updated edition in August 2008, it is commonly handed out by EEG practitioners around the world as a resource for their patients.

It begins, more or less, with Robbins saying that when he began his research, he "associated it vaguely with the seventies, the Beatles, and transcendental meditation. [It] had a New Age whiff about it. Add the words 'brain wave' and it sounded even wackier." But as he learns what EEG can do, he comes to find it "powerful, often beyond belief."

I stayed up until 3 A.M. finishing the book one night, high-lighting paragraph after paragraph, awestruck by Robbins's de-scriptions of how EEG training helped with everything from mental disorders to epilepsy to migraines to fibromyalgia—and how, unlike drugs, the results of EEG training were permanent. Too excited to sleep even when I did finish, I'd had what Rob-bins calls "the 'aha' moment." He writes, "The 'aha' moment will come when we as a culture realize we have a great deal of control over our nervous system and accept that responsibility. There is no reason for humankind to suffer from widespread anxiety, de-pression, ADD, ADHD, chronic pain, or a host of other ills."

The book is a bit dated now, but after reading it, I called Rob-bins, and he said that it all still holds up. The only difference now is that the tech is more affordable.

EEG's problem isn't just an unfortunate reputation, however:

it's that it seems to be something of a redheaded stepchild in the scientific community. A lot of scientists are dogmatically opposed. When Robbins writes that it is powerful beyond belief, this is literally true for many scientists. He means that in some cases, cynical scientists don't believe that the results are really as powerful as people claim.

Most of the evidence that EEG training works is "anecdotal"—simply the stories of people who've used something and say it worked for them. Scientists in general don't care for anecdotal evidence, viewing it as maybe a decent data point and possible reason to research something further, but nothing worth staking a reputation upon. (Not helping matters is that when people start talking about how powerful this can be, their language drifts toward the vernacular of evangelists.)

EEG is a difficult method to test according to modern standards for scientific rigor. This is the problem its skeptics have: not that EEG is dangerous or ineffective, but that they can't test it as simply as they can a pill. The most trusted research undergoes a third-party randomized double-blind placebo-controlled study. That means that some people get the actual product, or treatment, while some people get nothing, while yet others get a fake product or treatment—and nobody, not even the researchers, knows who's getting what until the end of the trial. "Third party" means that whoever paid for and is conducting the test has no financial or other interest beyond research.

These studies usually take weeks, and can take months or even years. They are expensive and difficult to carry out, so often companies first conduct their own tests to prove a drug works, then hope someone else will take interest and do a study, too.

And the short of it is that creating such a test for EEG training is virtually impossible. There is no sugar pill version.

So to put it mildly, EEG training is controversial. Some who say EEG training works say it works *too* well. But those like Dan Chartier, who have seen it not only change but save lives, don't worry about the skeptics. Harvard neurologist Dr. Frank H. Duffy has said that if a pill was as effective as EEG, "it would be universally accepted."

The way Robbins describes EEG training struck me as a vital lesson for anyone, athlete or otherwise. He writes, "Most human beings . . . are simply not inherently or irrevocably flawed. Instead, many—perhaps most—of the problems that plague humankind are a case of 'operator error.' We 'own' our central nervous system to a far greater degree than we imagine. We can get our hands on the steering wheel and deal with anxiety, depression, ADD, and a range of other problems. Neurofeedback shows us how powerful we are."

And now athletes are putting that to the test.

Chapter 3

"Holy Hell! This Is So Exciting!"

Sometime in mid-2010, Dr. Leslie Sherlin was at the Red Bull High Performance headquarters in Santa Monica, sitting in a meeting with none other than Andy Walshe. They were talking about Sherlin's company—then called Neurotopia, now called SenseLabs—that was working on using EEG training to help athletes.

"So," Walshe said, "if I have someone who's functioning very poorly, I can help them be healthy, or normal, whatever that means?"

"That's right," Sherlin said.

"All right, all right. Then what could you do for someone *already* performing at a high level? Can you make them even better?"

This hadn't even occurred to Sherlin. There's no way to know for certain, but Walshe might have been the first person in sports, maybe even the world, to think of using EEG not only as a powerful healing tool, but as a performance enhancer. Sherlin told

Walshe that he didn't know if that would work, but if Walshe was game, he wanted to try.

SenseLabs' three-story office building sits in the middle of an office park in the middle of town, surrounded by the rusty Arizona desert; Sherlin, who lives and works in Mesa, is a thoughtful man with a shaved head and runner's build.

Sherlin stumbled into this work back in college. After half-heartedly dreaming of becoming a musician and drifting around a few different undergraduate programs, he landed in psychology and found himself captivated by a class called Biological Basis of Behavior, where he learned to connect why people act and feel and think the ways they do with their brain activity. As he puts it, "People can stop fighting these battles in the wrong places."

When Sherlin met with Walshe in 2010, he knew of *some* research involving EEG and athletes, and a few folks around the country were trying it out, "but most of that work was still just sports psychology," he says. "Performance was not a big emphasis."

Soon after that fateful meeting, Sherlin installed an EEG setup—similar to the one in Chartier's office—in the Red Bull performance lab. Cap, computer, big monitor, all that. One of his coconspirators in this project was Dr. Michael Gervais.

Sherlin was nervous. His postdoctoral research had been in sports psychology, and he'd found it next to impossible to get athletes to even *talk* about their minds. And now, before they even had enough data to begin *guessing* whether EEG could help athletes, they *first* had to convince those scared men and women not just to talk about their minds, but to let them, in essence, hook their brains up to a computer. It doesn't get much more weird, intimate, and frightening than that.

But Sherlin severely underestimated the willingness of athletes to try pretty much anything that might make them even a little bit better, and it seemed that there was something appealing to them about the raw physicality of the process. Take, for instance, an Olympic sprinter Sherlin worked with—we'll call him John—who did great in practice and smaller events, but "just collapsed" in major competitions. Clearly, John's problem was mental, but he wanted nothing to do with psychology. The very topic upset him. But when he got his EEG assessment from Sherlin, he thought it was the greatest thing he'd ever seen, taking the report to his coach and saying, "Here's how my brain works!"

Of course, Sherlin's report displayed everything John's coach had been trying to get him to talk to a psychologist about.

Sherlin says, "It was like he said, 'I'm not gonna talk about the way I think or feel, but I'll talk about how my brain's working.' Even though they are the same thing."

When Gervais started working with the Seahawks, he connected them with Sherlin. Seahawks coach Pete Carroll, immensely interested in matters of the mind, wanted in. They gave everyone on the team an EEG assessment. The details are highly confidential, but there are good reasons for the Hawks' newfound obsession with meditation, mindfulness, and the like afterward.

What proved so powerful for the Seahawks and many other athletes Sherlin worked with was simply getting a visual of their brain in action. "There's real power in just connecting brain and body," Walshe says. "And when you see your brain on TV, in front of you, there's a 'holy shit' moment. What I think and how I feel and how I act are all related, and I can visually see it."

As athletes started getting into it, however, Sherlin, Gervais, and Walshe had a new challenge: finding language athletes could actually use. Sherlin would take their EEG and say something like, "Okay, you have *excessive theta* in the *dorsal lateral prefrontal cortex*. That means you're probably not going to be able to make decisions as well in moments of high stress."

The athlete would go, "Yeah, yeah, that's me! That makes sense!"

Then they'd leave, and their wife or husband or coach or trainer would ask, "Well, what'd you learn?" And they'd say, "I—I don't know. Too much of something, somewhere, in the something or other."

They recognized what Sherlin said about them, but they couldn't quite understand what it meant or what to do about it. "So," Sherlin says, "we were like, 'Okay, we've gotta change this.'"

They developed language that athletes latched on to more naturally, using terms such as *focus endurance, focus capacity, impulse control, decision-making capacity.*

As a result, even though it is dealing with the same fundamental psychological aspects of being an athlete, EEG doesn't *feel* like sports psychology because while it does, technically, deal with *feeeeeelings,* the approach is framed as, "How does my brain contribute to my performance?"

EEG data unties *feelings* from something *physical,* giving athletes, in essence, an objective way to examine and discuss their emotions. They can talk about the brain same as they talk about their muscles. Sherlin says, "It's not a muscle per se, but it behaves like one. So, how is your brain doing? How are we going to condition it? How will we strengthen it?"

In 2008, Olympic beach volleyball superstar Kerri Walsh Jennings and her partner, Misty May-Treanor, won gold at the Beijing Summer Olympics. That was Walsh Jennings's second gold medal. But then, in 2009, she watched as, in her words, her life "fell apart." She was married to a fellow volleyball player, and she was pregnant with their first child—but she was constantly on edge, or distracted, or otherwise not a good version of herself, and the result, she says, is that she and her husband were "on the verge of walking away from each other."

Telling this story in late 2014, she said, "I had this beautiful life, and on paper, I had everything I ever wanted, but I wasn't living my life, and I wasn't enjoying it."

A friend of hers told her about Mike Gervais, saying, "I called him for help with volleyball, but he helped me with my life."

So Kerri called Gervais, and, she says, they worked hard for two years. "We did a lot of work," she said. "And he . . . helped me find myself and get out of my own way, as an athlete, and as a woman."

In 2011, about fifteen months before the 2012 summer games in London, Gervais said Kerri should try Neurotopia. "And anything Gervais says for me to do," she said, "I will do until I die."

She got all hooked up in more or less the same way Dan Chartier hooked me up. "The gel actually improved my hair," she said. "So I was grateful for that."

Then she did her assessment test, which for Neurotopia was a twenty-minute continuous performance test consisting of tapping a touch screen when a dot appeared. That's it. The whole time she went through an entire range of emotions, everywhere from saying to herself *I'm kicking butt!* to *I'm failing!*

When she finished, she got her brain map, which Neurotopia produced differently from how Chartier did mine. Since they were trying to connect with athletes like her, instead of giving her several different views of a brain all lit up in reds and blues, she received a large hexagon-shaped graph with ten rings, resembling a target. Each point of the hexagon was labeled— *Activation Baseline, Stress Regulation, Max Activation, Impulse Control, Focus Endurance, Focus Capacity*—and scored on a scale of one to ten. The scores were indicated by a dot on the corresponding line of the ring, with better scores landing farther from center. A line connected each dot, creating a vivid picture of her brain.

Kerri's reaction was, in her words: *"Holy hell! This is so exciting!"*

In some ways, Kerri's EEG performance was amazing. For instance, the fastest a human brain *should* be able to process visual stimuli is about three hundred milliseconds, and yet Walsh Jennings's *average* response times were even faster than that—and she made few errors. She was also great at focusing and then sustaining her focus.

However, one area of her map cratered inward, almost creating the appearance of a brain in collapse. "First of all," Kerri said when she saw that, "am I gonna die? What *is* that? Why does my brain do that?"

Her two problem areas were activation baseline and stress regulation. To explain, Gervais told her, "You're a Ferrari . . . You go sixty to one-twenty. And you stay at one-twenty. You pull up to your house, pull into your garage, put it in park, and your foot is still on the gas, pedal to the metal, even in park."

In other words, although her brain was excellent at focusing and working hard, this came from a constantly high level of brain activity that in turn worked against her when she needed to, say, go home and relax. A common problem for people striving for high performance.

"And I go, 'Oh my God, that's exactly how I feel every day,'" Walsh Jennings said. "I feel like I'm burning the candle at both ends. I feel like I'm going too fast, especially when I get in an uncomfortable situation."

To see it on a screen like that snapped something in Walsh Jennings. She said, "My brain works this way because it thinks it's working perfectly, but it's not. I can change it. I can train it like it's a muscle."

Getting used to the training took some time. She sat in a chair with electrodes that were hooked into a computer attached to her head, looking at a big computer monitor, flying a ship through space with her mind. When she calmed her brain enough, the spaceship flew well. She felt like she was getting punked at first, but she committed to and trusted it.

At home, with her family, she learned to actually be there when she was there. Her relationship with her husband improved. Life began to *feel* as beautiful as it looked on paper.

The 2012 London Olympics came with Kerri facing her share of challenges. Not only was she thirty-three years old, entering that era of life when athletes' bodies begin working against them rather than for them, and not only had she given birth to her first child about a year earlier—she was also five weeks pregnant.

And yet, tall and dominant as ever, she and her partner, Misty May-Treanor, cruised to their third gold medal in as many Olympic appearances, losing just a single prelim set along the way. Kerri said, "I felt like I was a different athlete."

Meanwhile, despite success stories like Kerri's, Leslie Sherlin was realizing a fairly obvious problem: most of the world's elite athletes do not, in fact, live in Mesa, Arizona, or Marina del Rey, or Santa Monica. They might come by the office if they happened to be in town or lived nearby, but Sherlin saw a need for something they could use on their own—and something less clinical and intimidating, too, while he was at it. He envisioned people popping something onto their heads that they could simply use with their smartphones and tablets.

That took a long time. Taking clinical-grade technology and converting it into a consumer-ready product was a laborious process, to say the least. The hardware took forever to figure out, then they had to find a way to integrate this into a comfortable headset and package it all into something that someone could just put right on and start using. "It was a shit show," Sherlin says.

But Sherlin and Neurotopia pressed on, working on the design into 2012. The concept eventually evolved into a five-sensor EEG reader combined with Beats headphones that had EEG software built into them. They called it the BrainSport.

One of their first clients was an organization you might not immediately think of when it comes to elite athletes, but do they ever have, and need, elite athletes: the United States Department of Defense. The military loved the device, or at least the promise of it, for all the same reasons athletes do now.

Sherlin and his team kept working, and in 2013, the company shifted focus. "We just weren't getting the acceleration we wanted," Sherlin says. Their emphasis turned almost exclusively to *just ship a product.* Sherlin says this was "a major shift." "Before," he says, "it was teams, organizations, Department of Defense. This was a new consumer model."

They redesigned the BrainSport again by nixing the Beats headphones and creating their own, and they overhauled the hardware integrating the EEG. They also stopped shipping their clinical equipment to teams, and they pulled back from working with clients at Red Bull and in Gervais's office in Southern California. They knew they *could* help athletes with their clinical-grade equipment, which they didn't stop using completely, but they channeled their energy into the product. If they could crack a good, reliable, user-friendly headset, it would be one of the most powerful innovations to come along in a long time—not only for the world's elite athletes, but the world itself.

It took them until late 2013 to develop a workable prototype, which they kept fine-tuning throughout the year. Along the way, they rebranded and changed the company name from Neurotopia to SenseLabs, and the name of the product from BrainSport to Versus. You, versus your brain.

And finally, toward the end of 2013, they cracked it. They created something that worked. It has big, over-the-ear, gray headphones with a big neon-green headband—plus a second piece of headband that goes not side to side, but front to back. The headband has five sensors, each with fifteen small rubber prongs, and a clip dangling from the left earpiece. All of the EEG-reading hardware is built into the headset; the software comes from a downloadable app.

Sherlin and SenseLabs spent the first half of 2014 testing prototypes and fine-tuning some more before their consumer launch later that year. To celebrate, in November 2014, they held the SenseLabs Human Performance Council, inviting several athletes and leaders in sports psychology and neuroscience to discuss the future of performance training. Since 2011, numerous athletes at the top of their sports have begun training with SenseLabs and are now using Versus with success, in all different sports. To name a few: MLB all-star Carlos Quentin, NBA all-star Kyle Korver, six-time Winter X Games gold medalist and world record holder Levi LaVallee, world number-one-ranked doubles tennis player and fifteen-time Grand Slam titleholder Mike Bryan, Olympic gold medal-winning swimmer Eric Shanteau, and more in volleyball, golf, and various extreme sports.

Dr. Michael Gervais and Kerri Walsh Jennings went to the council, and at one point, Kerri took the stage before a crowd of about a hundred or so. She spoke in awestruck tones about what SenseLabs was doing. "I'm not paid to be here," she said. "I'm just a fan. But this is a big deal to me." She said another attendee had told her that athletes and other peak performers were trying to keep things like Versus hidden, but, she said, "I want to shout it from the mountaintops . . . I want you guys to know how life changing this can be."

Then she told her personal story. She said, "I think we all think we're stuck in this rut, and when we hit a rut, we're stuck there, but that's just nonsense. We need to take ownership of where we're at . . . And this is gonna allow me to do that [and] to kick butt in life."

After that, in August 2016, Walsh Jennings went to the Rio Summer Olympics. By then, she was thirty-seven years old, she'd had her *third* child, and her right shoulder was thoroughly taped—she'd dislocated it twice the summer before, and she had surgery in September 2015 to repair a torn labrum and capsule, the fifth surgery on that shoulder in her career. *And* she had a new partner, April Ross. And . . . they medaled all the same, taking home bronze.

About two weeks before I return to Chartier to get my EEG results—and learn what was so *interesting* about my brain—I get a delivery: my own SenseLabs Versus headset. (They were sold out, so Sherlin sent me an older prototype.) And because I'm impatient, instead of waiting for Chartier's results, I immediately take Versus for a spin.

The Versus app walks me through the necessary steps—charge the headphones, turn them on, hook them up.

The headset also comes with a small container of sensor gel, which goes on each sensor and the ear clip.

When I put the headset on, the app tells me how well each sensor is reading what it needs to read. Then the app starts my assessment. This is basic: a twelve-minute "game" that's called a "continuous performance task." This is, literally, nothing more than tapping the screen when a dot appears. That's it. If this sounds tedious and boring and kind of exhausting, well, it really is.

As I play the game, the EEG sensors collect my brain waves, which the software records. When I'm finished, the app instantly gives me an EEG assessment.

On the iPhone, this appears as a bar graph breaking down six categories: *activation baseline, focus capacity, impulse control, focus endurance, max activation,* and *stress regulation.* (The iPad app displays these results as the spider graph that Kerri Walsh Jennings saw back in 2011.) This is the Versus version of what Sherlin might see as an EEG clinician, reframed for athletes: instead of saying, for instance, that your brain is *generating too much beta in the occipital lobe,* which can indicate anxiety and stress, the program says that you are struggling with stress regulation. Or, if you're *generating too much theta in the frontal lobe,* you may have trouble with focus.

Of course, if an athlete, or anyone, has serious mental problems, they need clinical intervention—but for an athlete or whoever else wants a quick look at their brain and a way to shore up some weaker parts, this is astonishing, especially compared to what I went through in Chartier's office. Andy Walshe says that when they do their clinical EEG assessments at Red Bull, they have to outsource the analysis to a third party because it's so difficult to break down. And yet the Versus software does this instantly. Then it will, just as instantly, tell me where I need improvement—in focus or in stress. It automatically creates a training program, one twenty-minute session per day.

Working my way through the assessment, as I tap tap tap away at the flashing dots, that's where my mind goes, drifting into all sorts of thoughts about the Versus. I'm excited because the promise of it is enormous. The Versus isn't perfect—the sensors get painful after twenty minutes and leave indentions in your skin for more than a few minutes once you're finished—and the software could be a little better explained, but those feel like quibbles compared to seeing my brain on my phone.

That said, I'm skeptical, and I keep wondering, *How accurate can it be, really?*

When I finish my assessment, the results Versus gives me do not allay my skepticism. I'm already pretty certain that because of my anxiety and OCD, the Versus should tell me that I have problems with stress regulation, and maybe impulse control, although I expect to be pretty good at activation baseline, max activation, and focus—but the Versus app tells me my problem isn't stress at all. My problem is focus, and that's the training program it gives me.

For training, I literally play video games that I control with my mind. I fly a hot-air balloon, then I fly a glider, then I race a car around a track, then I play golf. Five minutes each. In the lower left-hand corner are three small circles. The better I focus, the more the circles converge, and the higher the hot-air balloon goes, the better the glider flies, the faster the car goes, and the more accurate and strong my golf shots are. If—when—I have too much trouble, the circles fly apart, and the game pauses itself to offer guidance. Breathe like so, avoid thoughts like such, focus on this part of the game, etc.

It's cool. And *hard*. When I'm done with my first twenty-minute session, I feel like I've finished a workout. But for several hours afterward, I feel more relaxed and, yeah, more focused. But this is strange. After all, I've been *clinically diagnosed* with anxiety and OCD. And the more I think about it—my OCD kicking in hard—the more it seems like maybe the Versus is too good to be true.

So, a couple weeks later when I'm back in Dr. Dan Chartier's leather chair, I'm dying to know: "OK, what was so *interesting*?"

"Well," he says, "people have told you that you have problems focusing before, correct?"

Wait. What?

I laugh. "No, actually. I thought that was the opposite of my problem."

He chuckles with me, being nice, but clearly confused. "Okay, then. Well, look at this."

On his computer, Chartier pulls up his brain-mapping program and opens my files. Several circles appear on the screen, most of them swathed in an array of pinks and oranges and reds. Not all of them. Some are clear. Healthy. But some also remind me of the planet Mars, others of Jupiter.

The good news, Chartier tells me, is that none of the blows to my head over the years seem to have done any permanent damage. The other news is, boy, do I have stuff to work on.

My theta waves (the lower-end ones associated with sleepiness and daydreaming and the like) were way stronger than they need to be. Same for my alpha waves (a level higher than theta) and my beta waves (the level above alpha) during tasks that require concentration and thought. Chartier explains that pretty much whatever is going on, I'm thinking about it all way harder than "normal"—hence the too-high beta waves. This could explain my anxiety and OCD. However, he seems even more concerned about how frequently my brain waves suggest that I drift into thinking about other things, too—he sees that because of the heightened theta. In other words, he says, I have a hyperactive imagination and daydream way too much.

For instance, my maps show enormous amounts of theta activity during a task involving math. Chartier says, "It's like your brain goes, 'Oh shit. MATH. Let me go think about something else.'" Same for a really boring, tedious reading sample written in ancient Queen's English. "Your brain found other ways to use its energy."

As we talk about all of this, we inevitably fall down the rabbit hole of my past. What previous therapy and research have taught me about my mind lines up with what Chartier is showing me on the screen, in regard not only to baseball, but to life. Everything we experience, particularly as children, shapes how our brains process information. In my case, I coped with stress by letting my imagination run wild with ways to make the stress could go away, in ways sometimes pragmatic and sometimes fantastical. "If we want to put it in a more *positive* way," Chartier says, "you're a *'creative'* person. And your ability to think outside the box is very important to you. You could think of your enormous theta waves as thinking *well* outside of the box—where, really, you're probably more like, *What box?*"

"There is no box!"

"Right. In a highly theta-driven brain, there is no box."

There's no question I have anxiety and OCD, Chartier says. But what this EEG assessment means is that many times, they are made worse by all of that outside-the-box thinking. It's great when I need to write or otherwise think creative thoughts, but a huge drag for everyday life. This plays out in different ways for people with OCD, and for me, I involuntarily imagine a million possible futures. In particular—when I was playing baseball, for instance—I constantly saw all the ways my life would be ruined by a mistaken decision. All that imagining exacerbates anxiety and obsessiveness.

Chartier hooks me back up to the computer. We don't have to use the whole cap now, and there is no *abrading*. He uses two sensors—one for the front of my skull, another for the back.

He pulls up a video game, a flyover of what looks like cinematic western scenery. Canyons, rivers, forests, that sort of stuff. When I concentrate—when I suppress my theta waves—I fly along. When I get bored and start to daydream—which happens, like, every two seconds—I slow down or stop completely. I do best when I put myself in a mind-set of relaxed control—not *straining*, but working, feeling zoned in but calm, thinking only of moving forward.

We do five sessions of five minutes each. And by the end of it, I am *beat*.

Chartier tells me that since the Versus's results were accurate, I can use it for training, and maybe check in with him every month or so if I want. That's the plan moving forward.

"And look, that's all we really promise," Chartier says. "There's nothing magical or mystical about this. This is no silver bullet. But what it can be is a road map—it's a GPS for your conscious-ness. It's not going to drive you where you want to go, but it's telling you, are you driving in the right direction?"

Afterward, I feel good. Focused without trying to be. On the drive home, I still feel normal pressures of life—work deadlines, frustration over wanting to spend more time with my family and friends, all that—and then someone cuts me off in traffic . . . but I'm calm. Normally, I probably cuss into the windshield, but to-day I just go, "Duuuuuuude, come on."

The days go by and that feeling fades. This is normal. Most people need at least thirty sessions to get lasting effects from EEG training. Some, even more. And even then, a tune-up every now and then. At first, I think I'll just bang those thirty out on the Ver-sus in a month and see where I'm at. That's not quite what happens. Over the next few months, I train when I can, sometimes on the Versus, sometimes on other tools that we will get to soon, some-times with Chartier. And it is *work*. That might be another reason why EEG training hasn't caught on. It's easy to pop a pill and see what happens, but EEG training feels almost like going to the gym.

Now, of course, the Kerri Walsh Jenningses of the world can't say that EEG training is the *only* reason they are great, and EEG won't have as dramatic an impact on everyone who uses it. Also, I hope this goes without saying, but to be clear: I'm not endorsing the approach of any single company—my goal here, as with all of This Stuff, is exploring what's possible and figuring out where we can learn more.

All that said, for people looking for an edge, something like EEG is seductive. It promises control over the mind in ways most of us would never think to imagine, offering a way to see our brain and then take action upon it.

So yeah, to borrow from Mrs. Walsh Jennings, holy hell, this is so exciting, indeed.

That's why I'm glad I talked with Dr. Pierre Beauchamp, a sports scientist based in Montreal, who provides a nice counterpoint. He has worked with elite athletes the world over, and he has substantial reservations about EEG training.

"Some people may have an imbalance in the brain, and it may be working for you," he says. "It may be why you're such a driven athlete, for instance. So if your neurofeedback specialist decides to change that imbalance, and says, 'You're going to be more optimally functioning,' and you go from top ten in the world to sixty-four in the world because your brain isn't operating the same way, you have to refigure it out. Is he doing performance enhancement, or is he doing clinical intervention?"

"Wait," I say. "So what you're saying is that if you were to balance somebody's brain out, you might actually *hurt* them as a performer?"

He nods.

So EEG could improve someone's quality of life, but Beauchamp says that that might not mean making them a better athlete—and it might even make them a *worse* athlete.

I ask Dan Chartier about this later. He says he's heard that argument before, but that it doesn't account for the deep work that he's seen EEG do for people. "The goal is to find flexibility," he says. "You want to be able to use what they call an 'imbalance' when you need it, but you want to also be able to slip out of that when you need to go about your day-to-day activities, and live your life outside of performance, too."

In the future, it may well be routine for an athlete to hook his or her brain to a computer (or some other sort of brain-analysis device) same as they go to the gym. But long before that happens, there is more to know about how the brain and the mind work.

What Chartier and Sherlin have shown me is invaluable, but the brain is the most complex object in the universe. There is a lot going on in there that we don't yet know about. The good news, however, is that we do know a lot more than we used to. And to know what's going on in our heads, we don't even have to have someone hook our brains to a computer.

Chapter 4

Home of the Mind

Let's revisit the comeback by Russell Wilson and the Seahawks from chapter one, specifically that wild two-point conversion. From the snap, to the play breaking down, to the wild scramble to keep the play alive, to finding his tight end and throwing him a pass he could score on, Wilson's brain was probably working as close to perfectly as possible.

I'll use this play as a way to explore what this means, and as a way to make sense out of the inner workings of the athlete's brain. Why? "It all comes back to being more aware," says Dr. Michael Gervais. "You need to be grounded and present, so that when you begin to do the thing that you're working on refining, you can have *conviction*, and you can have strength, and you can be fluid enough to adjust. So really, the very important variables are awareness and presence."

And the more aware you are, the better you are at being present. The reason why is a small structure in our brain partially responsible for predicting the future, called the "insula." This might be an oversimplification, but the insula is responsible for how we *feel* what we are experiencing. It processes an extraordinary amount of data, far more than we can process consciously. Our "gut feelings" are, in a sense, our processing of that data. Thus, the stronger our insula, the more we understand our experiences, and the more we can prevent our emotions from hijacking us and, say, hurling us into a blind rage or freezing us with fear.

Like everything else in the brain, with some work, the insula can be made stronger, not unlike a muscle. The more aware we are of what's happening around us—and within us—the more we can anticipate what might go wrong, meaning that when something does go wrong, we can better adapt, and thus be more successful.

That is how, say, Seahawks wide receiver Doug Baldwin came to have a working knowledge of things like *prefrontal cortex,* the frontal lobe in the brain, responsible for our ability to comprehend the future and plan for it. This is the last part of the brain to become fully active, by the way. In women, the prefrontal cortex may not be fully active until their early twenties or so—and in men, it can take until their later twenties. (This helps to explain the recklessness of so many young men and young folks in general—they literally might lack the physical tool they need to comprehend consequences, to truly grasp the meaning of "the future.")

Even a rough working knowledge of how the brain functions can have a powerful impact on someone's psyche. It creates, if not a sense of control, at least an awareness of why something might be happening. So, as for the rest of the brain, let's take a quick look. What's going on in the brain is complex, intricate, and fragile. That's why much of This Stuff exists—to help it all work as well as possible.

First, the brain falls into a few basic sections. There's the *brain stem,* which connects the brain and the spinal cord. This regulates our breathing, heartbeat, and blood pressure.

Then there are our three brains. Yes, "The Brain" is a collective of brains: as part of the brain stem, there's the *hindbrain,* taking up about the lower fifth of the overall brain. This automatically monitors body movements, keeps bodily processes in balance (such as respiration, circulation, and digestion), and so on. There's the *midbrain*—also part of the brain stem—a smallish chunk wedged above the hindbrain; this handles the more basic, automatic aspects of our vision, posture, and movement. Finally, the *forebrain,* which surrounds the midbrain, fills out the rest of the brain. This handles our higher functions, and this is what separates us from animals—the forebrain of humans is far more advanced than that of any other species.

The forebrain will be our primary focus.

Within the forebrain, we have the *cerebral cortex,* the uppermost, outermost layer of the brain, and the outermost layer of the *cerebrum.* This is where our *gray matter* grows. Its color comes from neural cell bodies.

The cerebral cortex is of a brilliant design, with layers upon layers of wrinkles folded on top of each other. This provides the cortex a vast surface area, and thus more neurons. This is also the part of the brain divided into left and right sides, split down the middle, and bridged by a thick bundle of axons in the center, called the *corpus callosum.*

Next, within the cerebral cortex, several different areas manage crucial parts of how we not only perform, but how we experience life. Over the course of my research I came to think of them as tiny people living in different regions of the brain, running the whole organ like a command center, an enormous network connected by a billion wires and in a constant swirl of communication, sending information back and forth and up and down to one another in nanoseconds. Some compare the brain to a machine; others say it's less like a machine (or a spaceship full of tiny brain people) and more like a quantum computer.

Whatever metaphor you like, the point is, the whole operation needs to be efficient and harmonious. All these tiny brain people have specific jobs, but they don't operate alone like engineers in separate offices—and really, the whole brain is, more or less, always doing something. The key players of any given moment need to be able to do their jobs without interference from the others.

And that's the goal at the heart of This Stuff: help the brain work *not* at *full blast,* but rather at maximum efficiency. This is necessary for all athletes—for all of us, really—but especially so for the NFL quarterback. Dr. Jeffrey Nicholl, a neurologist at Tulane, in 2010 told the *New Orleans Times-Picayune* that NFL quarterbacks needed the same, if not more, brainpower as, say, rocket scientists and brain surgeons. "You have to integrate all that you have learned into physicality," he said. "And such incredibly complex physicality, at that. The more I consider it, the more amazing it becomes."

On a related note: athletes, especially elite ones, have a natural leg up in brainpower for another reason, too. Exercise has been found to be a stunningly powerful tool for strengthening the brain. Working out sparks the release of serotonin, dopamine, norepinephrine, and endorphins, which play key roles in reducing anxiety and fighting off stress. Dr. Wendy Suzuki, a professor of neural science and psychology at the Center for Neural Science at New York University, in January 2016 wrote for *Quartz,* "That's why going for a run or spending 30 minutes on the elliptical can boost our moods immediately—combating the negative feelings we often associate with chronic stressors we deal with every day." Research Suzuki performed in her lab, published in November 2015 in the *Journal of the International Neuropsychological Society,* found that exercise helps people better shift and focus attention. She writes, "Even casual exercisers will recognize this effect. It's that heightened sense of focus that you feel right after you've gotten your blood flowing, whether it be a brisk walk with the dog or a full-on Crossfit workout. These findings suggest that if you have a big presentation or meeting where you need your focus and attention to be at its peak, you should get in a workout ahead of time to maximize those brain functions."

More amazing still, a September 2005 paper published in the *Journal of Neuroscience* said that studies of rodents indicate exercise improves memory because it boosts a process called "neurogenesis"—the birth of new brain cells.

Suzuki compares exercise to NZT, the drug that Bradley Cooper's character takes in the movie *Limitless* that takes him from slacker, loser writer to president of the United States.

Exercise literally makes the brain grow.

A group of researchers—led by Dr. Chris Eliasmith, a neuroscience professor and the director of the Centre for Theoretical Neuroscience at the University of Waterloo, Ontario—published a paper in *Science* magazine in November 2012 that provides a useful working paradigm for how the brain decides what to do. We'll use the Seahawks two-point conversion to walk through that.

The first phase in any athletic process is almost always *visual input,* meaning that from the start, as Wilson gets set behind the line of scrimmage, his *occipital lobe*—a big chunk responsible for vision that takes up most of the rear of the brain—is almost always firing away.

Then there's the matter of what to do with said input. That takes us to the *information-decoding* phase. Just above and in front of the occipital lobe, against the top rear to middle of our skulls, we have the *parietal lobe*. This handles how we perceive the world around us, as well as *spatial reasoning*, a critical aspect of almost every sport, and particularly useful when, say, seeing how close defenders are to you and your men, if you're Russell Wilson.

So, before calling "hike," Wilson glances over the defense, comparing what he sees to all those memorized schemes, deciding whether to audible. He draws from his *long-term memory*, managed by the *temporal lobe*—a fist-shaped piece of the lower, middle part of the brain, just above the brain stem and cerebellum—and performed by the *hippocampus*, a little seahorse-shaped fella within the temporal lobe.

Even before the game, Wilson's done a lot of work. Just to *start* a game as an NFL QB, you have to memorize some 120 to 150 plays, and not only know *your* jobs, but also the jobs of the other ten guys on the field with you, for each and every play. You also have to study film for about twenty to thirty hours a week so you know your opponent's defensive schemes—which usually number well into the dozens—so you know what to do against them, *and* you have to memorize how those schemes could change before *and* during a play.

Long-term memory draws from facts and memorization—concrete stuff—but also emotions. This is why fear can so directly lead to failure. This brings us to one of the stars of the show, "Migsby," the little peanut-shaped *amygdala* at the end of the hippocampus. Migsby will come up a lot more.

This is all part the *limbic system,* known as "the emotional brain," which manages all of our base needs: sensory processing and motor function (in the *thalamus*), emotion, thirst, hunger, circadian rhythms, body temperature, and control of the autonomic nervous system (the *hypothalamus*), memory, emotion, and fear (Migsby), and learning and converting short-term memory to long-term memory along with recalling spatial relationships in the world around us (the hippocampus).

At this point, Wilson's *working memory* kicks in, acting as the brain's scratch pad. Generally, we can log about seven things at a time—phone numbers, negotiation details, where defenders are lined up in the secondary—for about fifteen to sixty seconds. This takes place within another star, "Big Fronty," the *frontal lobe*, which will also come back up quite often.

This is all happening as Wilson simply stands at the line of scrimmage, by the way.

Just standing there, from front to back, his brain has gone to work—and that, only if he's calm. Wilson almost always is, which is why he's so good. When his teammates call him a robot, it's a compliment: robotic reliability and efficiency are what you want out of your quarterback's brain. When athletes panic in such situations, it's usually because they are thinking too much, often about how things could go wrong. *That* activates Migsby, a major influential player in the brain's fear network.

While he is still in shotgun, having surveyed the field, Wilson's brain completes the *information-decoding and transform-calculations* phase. In other words, the brain's made sense out of what he sees, and now figures out what to do about it. Next phase: *reward evaluation.* This one's simple. To start the play, Wilson needs to hike the ball.

Set. Hut. Hike.

Now Wilson has some of the biggest, strongest, fastest, scariest men in the world trying to get him, and he has about three seconds to process everything that happens next and decide what to do about it.

Information decoding starts again, breaking everything down and sending out responses. *Motor processing and motor output* ramps into overdrive. The whole process starts all over. The *motor cortex* links with the midbrain to drive Wilson's body around the field. Wilson moves smoothly, with no wasted effort, the result of countless thousands of hours of practice.

When the play breaks down—receivers covered, defenders breaking blocks and getting into his face, all that—Wilson's *pattern recognition* kicks in.

He scrambles.

The temporal lobe, which handles comprehension and harboring memories, sounds a red alert. *Everything's gone to hell—we gotta do something else or we are SCREWED!*

Big Fronty goes to work solving that problem.

A look into the brain here would show a breathtaking display of electricity and chemicals and energy.

Wilson doesn't panic. He examines the broken play, seeks a solution. He can do this, in large part, because of that insula. Clearly, Wilson's insula is a beast. He's seen this sort of thing hundreds of times before, sometimes in real life, but many times in his mind. Wilson spends time each week with his eyes closed, visualizing what can happen on the field, both good and bad.

Now, that ridiculous throw to his tight end. As he was scrambling away from the defense, Wilson couldn't have *consciously* thought to do that. To do amazing athletic things, Big Fronty—the "thinking" part of the brain—has to shut *down.* Actual *thought* takes a lot of time and energy, and the brain is in a constant state of competition with itself for resources.

In other words, all our little brain people *try* to be involved, but the ones trained to rise in certain situations will take control.

Having seen everything, when Wilson looks to throw, he doesn't question it, because he can't—he can only *turn and throw.*

That he was able to do that so unconsciously likely means his brain was operating at its full potential. He was on automatic.

We've all heard the myth about how we use only 10 percent of our brains. The truth is that our brains are generally running close to 100 percent—except for when, like Wilson in that moment, flow has taken over and we've gone automatic; in those moments, most of the brain actually shuts down, except for only the most necessary parts.

When Eminem raps about "lose yourself in the moment," there's scientific basis for that. On automatic, one of the primary parts of the brain that shuts off is the *neocortex,* which takes up most of the cerebral cortex. This is the part of the brain that makes mammals, and humans in particular, so unique. Birds and reptiles don't even have one, and it's huge in humans. With six different layers folded over each other, the neocortex is what makes human beings capable of complex thought. One of its primary jobs is imagining the future, a fantastic advantage for humans. This is also the part of the brain that causes us to all at once conceive of something like *infinity* and wrestle with the overwhelming questions of what that means for us.

And among other things, the neocortex is the part of us that is aware that we are "someone," that we have a "self."

In flow, the neocortex shuts down, and we forget about ourselves.

And so worries *about* ourselves disappear.

You know that inner critic that drives you crazy, the one always finding something wrong with whatever you're doing? That comes from Big Fronty, and is an ancient survival tool, keeping us in check. But as anyone with anxiety knows, the neocortex and that inner critic can combine to really mess us up.

On automatic, however, *hypofrontality* occurs, meaning that our frontal cortex *shuts down,* and that makes our inner critic shut the heck up.

In other words, we need our brains fired up in full to learn and prepare and train—but come game time, it's best to let go and trust our bodies to do what they need to do. When we lose ourselves, when we go automatic, then we can slip into an other-worldly mind frame of calm, focus, and perception. We know all and we fear nothing.

Chapter 5

The Problem and Inevitable Death of Stigma

"I wish the whole world could see what I see," the man standing at the edge of space said.

It was October 14, 2012, and this was Red Bull's Project Stratos. The mission: have a man leap from space, from higher than any human had leaped before, and land safely on earth, and break the sound barrier to go supersonic along the way. Wearing a space suit, Felix Baumgartner—the five-foot-seven Austrian skydiver, BASE jumper, and all-around daredevil nicknamed "Fearless Felix"—stood 128,100 feet above Earth. That's twenty-four miles. He'd just stepped to the edge of a small pod that, hours earlier, had launched from the Roswell International Air Center in New Mexico, lifted by massive helium balloon.

Several cameras mounted on the pod and in his helmet broadcast everything, live, around the globe. Eight million people were watching it live on YouTube alone. In a way, they *could* see what he saw: the planet in full, huge and round, a giant ball of life, impossible against the black darkness of space.

"Sometimes," Baumgartner continued, looking down at the planet, "you have to get up really high to understand how small you are. I'm coming home now."

Then he jumped.

Baumgartner fell for nearly four and a half minutes and reached a top speed of 843.6 mph. He broke the sound barrier. No other human has ever done that without an engine driving him.

But somewhere in the stratosphere, where the air is too thin to keep a falling object stable, Baumgartner went into a spin. Fifty-three years earlier, in 1959, the same thing had almost killed the one man who'd done this before, Air Force colonel Joe Kittinger, who dove from nineteen miles high. In 1966, Nick Piantanida tried to break Kittinger's record and died. There was good reason the record stood.

In Baumgartner's case, if he couldn't correct his spin in time, he'd lose control, eventually rotating with such speed that his blood would be sent away from the center of his body; if he went too fast, the only place left for the blood to go would be out of his eyes, which would mean his life was over.

He fought the spin. He didn't panic. He righted himself.

Moments later, the parachute deployed without fail, and he drifted to Earth and landed with a light jog, then fell to his knees and raised his hands.

I was one of the eight million people watching live on YouTube that day, and that was one of the most moving things I'd ever seen. There was something visceral about watching a man leap from space. But furthermore, during Baumgartner's ascent, I read up on him, and I realized that as amazing as his skydive from space was, his greatest accomplishment might have been reaching space at all.

Red Bull didn't announce Project Stratos until early 2010, but they'd been planning it for a while. From beginning to end, the whole thing took some five years.

Baumgartner made a name for himself as a daredevil who BASE-jumped off some of the world's tallest buildings, often illegally. He'd flown across the English Channel with nothing but a carbon-fiber wing. He earned the nickname "Fearless Felix." But at forty-three, as Red Bull was pouring $18 million into Project Stratos and Baumgartner was training for the jump, he freaked out. He later told journalist Donald McRae for the *Guardian,* "You and I know Fearless Felix doesn't really exist. He might seem like a cool guy, but I've had to address a real psychological battle. It's been way harder than stepping out into space."

Baumgartner wasn't scared of the jump itself and all that could go wrong during it. He wasn't scared of the fact that Piantanida had died trying the same jump about fifty years earlier. Jumping out of a plane or off a building or cliff was as easy as going for a walk—he'd been doing it for twenty-five years—but he'd been doing it in comfortable, light clothing. He was scared of the space suit. "When I skydive," he said, "even in winter, I wear very thin gloves. I want to be flexible, with fast reactions."

The suit was a monster, though—not flexible, thick gloves, twice as heavy as he was used to. He couldn't move his head very well. For instance, during a normal skydive, when he deployed the chute, he'd look up to make sure it inflated—but he couldn't do that wearing a space helmet. He'd have to put two mirrors on his gloves in order to check the chute. He couldn't even feel the air on his body, meaning he wouldn't know if he needed to make an adjustment until he was already in error.

His first test jump in the space suit, as he stood on the edge of a plane at thirty thousand feet—"It felt like my first skydive," he said. "The same fear from twenty-five years ago is back."

He could handle the suit for maybe an hour, on the ground. Anything beyond that, however, and claustrophobia crippled him. That was a big problem, because the balloon ride to space alone would take three and a half hours. Between that, and the prep time, and the dive itself, he was looking at five hours in the suit, minimum.

During training, Baumgartner got so stressed he couldn't sleep. The suit's rubber smell made him sick. Plenty of people tried to help, even the man whose records he was trying to break, Joe Kittinger himself, then eighty-four years old; he'd come on the project as chief adviser. Not even Mike Todd, Baumgartner's life-support engineer, could help him, and he was someone Baumgartner said felt like his own father. Baumgartner talked to a psychologist for the first time in his life—none other than Michael Gervais. Baumgartner's reaction to needing that kind of help was the same reaction that it seems almost everyone has: "It was so embarrassing."

One week in mid-2010, when Baumgartner was supposed to undergo an endurance test in the space suit, he decided, instead, to flee the country. He went back to Austria and took shelter in his home town of Salzburg. He was done. Later that year, in September 2010, he was arrested after a fit of road rage in which he punched a taxi driver and drove off, leaving the driver bloody.

Meanwhile, Project Stratos didn't stop. There was more to it than a cool stunt. They were working with project medical director Dr. Jonathan Clark, who'd overseen the medical needs of space shuttle crews at NASA, to test various aids for astronauts, such as space suits, escape concepts, and treatment protocols for pressure loss at extreme altitudes.

About six months after leaving Project Stratos, Baumgartner saw video of Red Bull testing one of the space suits. When he saw another man wearing it, he was jealous. *You're not supposed to be in my suit.*

Mike Gervais flew to Austria and spent some time with him. They did a lot of deep work, like self-talk, breathing techniques, and a method called "flooding," also known as "systematic desensitization," to drown the fear. Gervais also had Baumgartner talk to an imaginary son about what was happening to him. Baumgartner found it all, again, in his word, "embarrassing," but he also made his way back to America. He told the *Guardian* he also unpacked a key aspect of his claustrophobia: "It's not my fault. It's just in my mind."

Even then, he still had to convince the Red Bull team he could do it. Everyone doubted him, which shook him all the more. "I never thought Mike [Todd] would doubt me," Baumgartner said. "He was like my father . . . Nobody had faith in me anymore."

But Baumgartner learned to channel his anxiety into something productive. Instead of focusing on the horrors of the suit or the worries of the people he cared about, he focused on a moment beyond the fear, his ultimate goal: after he jumped from the pod, he wanted to go supersonic.

Come time to launch, Baumgartner had a team of three hundred people coordinating with him in a NASA-style mission control operation, including more than seventy engineers, scientists, and doctors. The last person he saw before stepping into the capsule was his man Mike Todd. "Okay," Todd said, smiling. "See you on the ground, buddy."

On his way to space, the visor on Baumgartner's helmet got foggy, and for a while they thought he'd have to do the jump half blind. Mission control almost called the whole thing off. Baumgartner's claustrophobia threatened to rise.

No, Baumgartner said.

They worked through it.

After he jumped, Baumgartner knew he was going to be okay. He went supersonic, the first human to break the sound barrier without an engine. And when he landed, he saw Mike Todd, smiling.

"The suit was my worst enemy," he said. "But it became my

friend. Because the higher you go, the more you need the suit. It gives you the only way to survive. I learned to love the suit up there."

Not everyone's problems are as extreme as surviving while trying to go supersonic during a twenty-four-mile free fall to Earth, but that's sure how they can feel.

Problem is, when it comes to anything mental, especially in sports, silence and secrecy have been the status quo. A certain taboo has surrounded such talk, suffocating like toxic smog.

Or, like a space suit.

Before anyone can do anything to make their minds better, they have to be willing to look at it and say there is a problem. For far too many people, that only happens after a long, hard fall.

The thought of saying it out loud—*"I need help"*—made me feel like my heart was clogging my throat. What scared me was being seen as weak or crazy. But the truth is, to quote Dr. Daniel Chao, founder of Halo Sport: "It's almost like it's easier to come out as gay now than to say you see a psychologist. We all know Jason Collins is gay, but we can't talk about the fact that pretty much any athlete at the elite level is seeing a therapist every week."

And the truth—maybe the most important, sobering truth—is that, as dramatic as my problems felt to me, they were *common*, and many people end up way worse. About sixty million Americans age eighteen or older have a diagnosable mental disorder, and nearly two billion people worldwide. That's 138 times the number of people who have cancer. Almost 25 percent of the human race, one out of every four of us, are suffering. And at least half of us never get help.

That's just the general population.

The truth is also that, among athletes, the situation is even worse.

In 2012, Dr. Lynette Hughes, a senior research officer at Compass Research and Policy, and Dr. Gerard Leavey, the director of research at Compass Research, published a paper in the *British Journal of Psychiatry* saying that athletes, of all ages and genders, suffer from mental illness at a much higher rate than the average population.

In October 2016, NCAA chief medical officer Brian Hainline told me, "Concussion may be the elephant in the room, but mental health is the single most important health and safety issue facing our student athletes."

A January 2016 report published in the *British Journal of Sports Medicine* found that about a quarter of all college athletes show symptoms of depression. One-third of all professional football players are estimated to have mental health issues.

Of course, concussion, and other brain damage, plays a large role. In 2014, researchers at Boston University dissected the brains of seventy-nine deceased NFL players to find that seventy-six of them contained evidence of *chronic traumatic encephalopathy,* or CTE. While this can be caused by severe blows to the head that result in concussions, it is also brought on by the smaller, more regular impacts football players suffer during their career. People with CTE frequently suffer memory loss and impaired judgment as well as depression. They also suffer terrible pain, both physical and emotional, leading to raging outbursts and suicide. One of the more horrific cases of CTE was that of Jovan Belcher, the Kansas City Chiefs linebacker who shot his girlfriend to death and then shot himself in 2012. CTE sufferers aren't limited to football either—in 2016, legendary BMXer Dave Mirra, after lunch with friends, went to his truck, pulled out a gun, and shot himself dead. One of the worst parts of CTE is that it's only diagnosable by brain dissection, meaning sufferers can never really know if they have it.

Beyond brain injury, Hughes and Leavey say that a big reason why athletes struggle so much with their mental health is simply because of the nature of aspiring elite athletes' lives. Their world demands enormous investments of time and energy, and it often drains them of not only their own free time, but also their very selves. In brief moments, this is a huge benefit—but what we're talking about here is that athletes, often without even realizing it, lose any sense of personal identity beyond their sport. Their entire existence serves their team and their sport, and they are often *told* what to do, rendering them impotent, rather than living with the freedom to make choices.

This leads to a condition Hughes and Leavey call "Identity Foreclosure," which is exactly what it sounds like—afflicted athletes *have no identity* beyond their sport.

Dr. Michael Gervais agrees that this is one of athletes' most common psychological pitfalls. They forget that they are human beings who need a life and personality beyond their sport. He calls this "the coupling of one's identity to one's performance."

I asked Gervais what this looks like in the physical brain, and he says we don't know yet. To take an educated guess, however, one could imagine this having to do with the *fight-or-flight* response becoming too active when one is challenged, or when one is struggling in sport. In the brain of someone who mistakes their performance for their very identity, it follows that a threat to successful performance is a threat to one's life.

One of the hardest things about keeping athletes healthy is that when an athlete mistakenly couples his identity with his performance, it can actually lead to impressive results at first. For me, and for those who suffer likewise, performance equals life, and so we work hard. This generates an intense drive and work ethic that many people admire—modern American culture, in fact, seems to idolize this sacrificing of life to work.

And for a time, it *can* be of benefit. For me, that meant working obsessively on everything from improving my swing to getting stronger and everything else. It can make you care deeply and drive you to fantastic results.

"At some point," however, Gervais says, "that becomes just a drain."

When the drain sets in—and it always does—it manifests itself as burnout, injury, insomnia, chronic fatigue. Athletes, male and female alike, are also highly prone to eating disorders and body dysmorphia. (For me, even at 220 pounds and 7 percent body fat, I'd look in the mirror and think I looked pudgy and soft.)

Perhaps one of the most visible ways we see athletes compensate for this sort of imbalance is in an outsized urge to take dangerous risks. Hard partying. Heavy drinking. Driving drunk. Having unprotected sex with strangers. And so on. Some people argue that athletes acting in dangerous ways are just people with character flaws or "just weren't raised right" or are "just boys being boys." And while that might be part of the problem, it's not a valid reason as often as people like to imagine. Hughes and Leavey, in their February 2012 paper in the *BJP*, make a compelling case that risky and/or aggressive behavior likely becomes more pronounced—in people prone to it—because of the nature of über-competitive elite sports.

For the best athletes in the world, virtually every aspect of their life is more or less dictated and scheduled in order to maximize how good they can be at . . . their game. And in the meantime, when they do work out, and when they do compete, they are reaching into the utter depths of themselves to pull the uttermost out of themselves.

It takes a certain willpower and high-intensity mind-set to do that, and frequently, as Kerri Walsh Jennings found, that's not a trait that is so easily turned on and off. To see when it is running away with your mind typically means a great deal of struggle first, and frequently that struggle means some sort of damage in one's life—and all of this adds up to unique, unnatural stress. That stress, in turn, can easily trigger risky, aggressive, strong impulses that, left untreated, can metastasize into something even more dangerous.

In short, at the very least, unless athletes conscientiously tend to their mind, sports can exacerbate their worst impulses.

To be clear: sports in and of themselves are not a problem for athletes' mental health. The problem is that sports have historically obfuscated and even demonized mental needs, and treated them as inherent weaknesses, when really they are issues that treatment often can resolve. Hughes and Leavey write, "Despite a number of high-profile breakdowns and tragedies among athletes, there remains a tendency among sports governing bodies and officials to downplay or ignore the significance of psychiatric symptoms."

They go on to say that sports' current approach to mental health is "fraught with stigmatization, denial, and dichotomous paradigms of 'psychological' versus 'physical' disease, which are inaccurate, unhelpful, and deprive the athlete of effective care."

Part of the problem, as they see it, is the nature of the "distorted or absent" relationship between athletes and team doctors: "Doctors working within the sporting environment are frequently under intense pressure from management, coaches, trainers, and agents to improve performance in the short term, and are therefore faced with a myriad of ethical dilemmas that compromise the well-being and treatment of the athlete."

Psychiatrist Janet Taylor recently told *New York Times* columnist William C. Rhoden, "Professional athletes are used to seeing themselves as warriors able to withstand multiple physical challenges, and have battled to get to the next level because of their mental and physical toughness. Now they may be sidelined by an enemy they can't even see: their mind."

Not every athlete who suffers Identity Foreclosure also suffers from narcissism, but the former can and frequently does breed the latter in sports.

Experts have identified three types of narcissism. One, the most "typical" type, is the grandiose, boastful man or woman openly vying for everyone's attention. Two, the "covert" narcissist, is more like I was (and still am some days), full of irrational fear and anxiety about how I appeared, perpetually trying to fight off the fear, either consciously or unconsciously. Then there's the "communal" narcissist, who bolsters their image by doing anything and everything they can "for others," when their true goal, even subconsciously, is projecting a certain image.

That's why sometimes über-talented types choke in critical moments—they are either consciously or subconsciously worried about how their failures will reflect on them, because they are more concerned with themselves, and with how they *appear*, than with the final outcome. Of course, *some* concern about self is natural and even healthy. It's when that becomes imbalanced that problems arise. People overly concerned with self, for instance, can be thrown off track by worries about how failure will affect them, which activates the part of the brain aware of the "self," which then derails everything else.

On top of all of this, there is also the ever-looming specter athletes face of catastrophic injury, or failure, or God only knows what else that could cost them their jobs. It takes a profound mental toll, considering that these men and women's whole lives and livelihoods depend upon peak performance. Athletes commonly react to an injury with the same level of emotional anguish and grief that most people feel at the death of a loved one; 20 percent of injured athletes warrant clinical psychological intervention, including for risk of suicide.

Alpine skier Picabo Street won the 1998 Winter Olympics Super G, and along the way, displayed a bold, spunky personality that captured the hearts of the world. Later that year, she crashed while skiing in Switzerland. It was horrific—she broke her left leg and blew out her right knee. In the months that followed, she later told the *New York Times,* she "went all the way to rock bottom," locking herself in a bedroom at her parents' house, closing the blinds and refusing to see anyone or answer any phone calls. She just lay there in the dark, literally and figuratively. She didn't even watch TV. "I went from being a very physical person, a very powerful athlete, to barely having any strength to get from my room to the kitchen," she said. "You're stuck, and you can't do what you normally do, and it makes you crazy."

Recovery, from both the physical injuries and the mental, took her almost two years.

And then there is the suffering athletes endure when their careers finally do end. Author John Feinstein once wrote, "Athletes die twice." He repeated this in 2012 during a radio interview while discussing the recent suicide of Junior Seau, the ten-time All-Pro, twelve-time Pro Bowl–selected linebacker who retired following the 2009 season, then killed himself in May 2012.

The death of an athlete's career, whether an all-star or a role player or a college kid who never quite got his shot, always feels like heartbreak, like the loss of one's world. Without knowing what's going on, and without a good support system, the fallout can be catastrophic. They know that there are more important things going on in the world, but try telling that to the heart.

"As an athlete," three-time NASCAR Winston Cup champion Darrell Waltrip told ESPN in the wake of Seau's death, "your identity is tied up in what you've done. It's your platform. So when that's taken away, you get a little nervous, scared about, *Where do I go from here?*"

Brad Daugherty, the number one pick in the 1986 NBA draft, said, "You lose that identity, and it goes away as soon as you hear the word 'former.' That word stings. So when you see what happens to guys like Junior Seau . . . I hate that it came to that, but a little piece of me understands it. That scares me a little bit."

And yet, for all the psychological peril athletes face, as difficult as it might be for the average person to talk about mental illness, it seems even more difficult for athletes. In early 2015, Duke women's basketball player Oderah Chidom told Fox Sports that student athletes viewed getting professional help with mental health as a "sign of weakness." She said, "No one wants to admit there's a problem until it's too late." ESPN staff writer Tim Keown, who's covered elite athletes for decades, recently wrote, "Mental illness remains a great unexamined and unacknowledged aspect of society in general and sports in particular. It cuts across social, racial, and economic boundaries, but it is misunderstood to such an incredible degree that a portion of the population questions not only its impact on an individual, but its very existence."

Wes Clapp, a cofounder of the Cambridge, Massachusetts–based company NeuroScouting, told me, "When you blow out your ACL, nobody's like, *Dude, you gotta go to a doctor for that!* It's like, of course. And it should be the exact same way, where you're like, *I either have something going on and want to get it checked out, or I just want to make sure.* Or even, *I could be spending more time refining everything. I spend just as much time in the gym—I should be trying to refine everything else, without that kind of stigma.* But you go to someone for mental help, and it's like, *Oh, why are you going there? Why are you talking to them?* It's seen as a weakness, which nobody associates with any other kind of medical issue."

Let's be clear: this isn't the case across the board, and things *are* shifting. Slowly, and so quietly it almost seems like a secret, but they are shifting. Michael Gervais says that the athletes he works with are all surprisingly comfortable talking with him about their mental needs. Several people have told me that most of the world's best athletes talk with sports psychologists or other therapists such as Gervais regularly—it's just that we haven't known about it.

There have been a few lights in this mental health wilderness over the years. Joey Votto, an all-star first baseman for the Cincinnati Reds, went on the disabled list for three weeks in 2009, and afterward revealed that he had been suffering severe depression and anxiety in wake of his father's death the year before. "I thought I was going to go crazy," he said. It became so severe that he was hospitalized twice. "I really hadn't acknowledged how important it is to express the things I had been dealing with on the inside," he told the Associated Press that June.

Brandon Marshall, the great New York Jets wide receiver, has openly talked about his own dealings with borderline personality disorder. Before he got help, it even landed him in jail. He and his wife started the nonprofit Project 375 to take on the stigma of treating mental health, not only at the elite level but throughout the world.

Ohio State football coach Urban Meyer touched on this briefly in 2014 for HBO, describing his addictive and obsessive struggles, then went deep into his problems with me in 2016 for a story for Bleacher Report's *B/R Mag*. He described a highly detailed, purposeful set of mechanisms he uses to keep his mind on track. (And even then, he says, he "drifts" off course about fifty times a day.) Meyer told me it's long past time that people started talking about all of this more openly. To that end, he detailed various mental battles of his own that he says he also knows many, if not most, great coaches struggle with. Anxiety. Depression. Obsessive-compulsive disorder. He laid out the ways they nearly destroyed his life, and the ways he's learned how to battle them. He learned one secret after another about how the brain works, and he has since become obsessed with finding ways to help not only himself, but also his coaches and his players, with mental health challenges.

Meyer also discussed at length the need for everyone to better communicate about mental illnesses. To that end, he doesn't even like using the term *illness*. Of course, there are people in the world who have hard-core, full-blown illnesses that need intensive psychiatric intervention and even hospitalization. But there is a spectrum to these things—on one end, say, asthma; on the other, a punctured lung. Both are, technically, breathing disorders. So when it comes to mental health, terms like *illness* and *disorder* alienate people, make them recoil, when really, all they might need is a metaphorical mental inhaler.

Meyer compares mental problems to physical injuries. "I never use the term *illness,* because I don't believe that," he says. "I believe it's no different than if somebody got a muscle pull. That's not a hamstring illness."

He calls it "getting the mind right." And he has made Ohio State University's football program maybe the most progressive elite NCAA program in the country when it comes to providing their staff and student athletes the tools necessary to (1) understand mental health and then (2) manage it properly. They have everything from sports psychologists on staff to regular, intensive, hours-long workshops.

All of this serves to foster those hard-to-start conversations about what it actually means to be mentally strong. And when people do start having those conversations, profound changes take place.

Take Oliver Marmol. He was a junior shortstop at the College of Charleston in 2007 when the St. Louis Cardinals drafted him. Five years later, they asked him to manage their rookie team in Johnston City, Tennessee, making him, at twenty-five, the youngest manager in baseball. "That just means I wasn't a very good ballplayer," he says with a laugh.

In practice, he was comfortable. Zero anxiety, played like a big-league shortstop. But then the game started, and boom: "Panic," he says. And it was like all the hard work he'd put in never happened.

Only when Marmol became a coach did he realize that tons of other guys were dealing with the same thing. "And," he says, "you learn not to talk about this at an early age, and to just deal with it."

We've all heard it—suck it up. Figure it out. Grin and bear it. "They sound motivating," Marmol says, "but it's a ton of crap, because at the end of the day, you will cave."

Marmol found his calling as a coach. His first year, they had a winning record, and the next season, he was promoted to manager of the State College Spikes, the Cardinals' short-season single-A minor league affiliate. They won the division title that year, and the league title the year after that. Then Marmol was promoted to their high single-A team, the Palm Beach Cardinals, where they went 75–63 and made a deep postseason run, falling in the semifinals.

Along the way, Marmol's perspective underwent a dramatic shift. As a player, he'd always felt a vague sense that the guys who *could* go out and play well were different, but he knew that they *all* felt butterflies, too, which, really, is just anxiety. But the good players handled those emotions differently. As a coach, he learned that it doesn't get processed as *anxiety* in their brains the way it does in brains like his and mine. He learned, "It doesn't create a panic in them. They use it to fuel what's about to happen."

Furthermore, it's one thing to suffer from that sort of paralyzing anxiety and maybe see it in teammates, as a player; as a coach, to see your players suffer like that is something else entirely. And yet traditional ways of coaching, when you start really thinking about them, have been—well, there's no polite way to say this. They've been willfully ignorant at best, moronic at worst.

When a player develops a problem—booting routine ground balls, developing the Yips, freezing at the plate—Marmol says, "The traditional idea has always been, 'Don't talk about it, because he's going to get worse.' That's not the answer. The player knows he has a problem. The coach knows he has a problem. But then there's this rule. *Let's not talk about it so it doesn't get worse.* And it's like, dude, it's serious. But there's always this divider, where the coach knows, and the player knows, but nobody talks about it."

End of the day, you will cave.

Marmol had enough. He said, "There has to be something more to this," and he dove into the research about, in his words, "the neuro side of things," with one main question driving him: "How do we start to train from the neck up?"

One of the first things he learned was also one of the simplest and most important: "The best in the world, they *have* those conversations."

Marmol managed several guys who went on to play in the majors, and several more who seemed well on their way. You know the type. They take care of themselves on *and* off the field, they seem locked in every day, all that. And Marmol realized that everything the rest of us are scared to talk about, those elite guys talked about.

"They have teams of people, and they have those conversations," he says. "And they make sure they're very open about all of these mental things. And because they don't have insecurity, they're able to handle things a lot better. It's all out in the open for them. They know they're the best, and they want to figure out, *Hey, how do I get better in these areas? If I'm not open about them, I can't improve them.* We just don't *know* about it, because we're not in those circles."

So he started just trying to start conversations with his players. It wasn't easy. "A lot of these guys—you gotta remember, we draft them, they're the hottest thing in high school or college," Marmol says. "And then they get into an arena where everyone's as good as them, and they can fake their way through it, as far as how they verbalize things to their managers or their staff, so they're never gonna open up about any of these insecurities. So the more we can start asking the right questions, and just being a little more up front, they'll start to open up."

To use anxiety as an example: when it takes over, a potentially destructive part of our brain is taking control. Parts of our brains are nearly identical to those of animals. There's the *cerebellum,* our "lizard brain," which runs our body almost unconsciously, and, when necessary, reacts nearly as unconsciously. When you fly into a fit of rage, or break down bawling, or feel like running away screaming, that's the cerebellum hijacking you. In fact, while many people believe that having an anxiety attack means curling into a ball on the floor, it can also mean many other things, including what may seem like a fit of rage.

No one yet knows *exactly* all the connections between the cerebral cortex and the cerebellum and the cerebrum, and the smaller parts within them, such as the insula, Migsby (the amygdala), and so on. However, we do know that Migsby is one of the brain's fear centers, and the insula plays a large role in the brain's anticipation of what's going to happen next, which, for obvious reasons, has a large impact on how much fear you feel. And it seems that the more fear you feel—the more Migsby gets worked up—the more your cerebellum takes over. In other words, the more afraid you become, the more your instinctual, animal brain takes over, rendering you even more incapable of acting with calm and intelligence.

The more you can overload that cerebellum—the more you can teach it about the world, in other words—the more you can train it not to freak out every time something out of the ordinary happens. Basically, train it not to interpret every unexpected, unknown, undesired event like the end of the world.

That said, there is the finest of lines between losing yourself in flow and losing yourself to fear. Flow and fear are close cousins. It's the athletes who channel fear into flow who have a greater chance of success.

Basically, you can't control fear. You can't force it away. That's because fear is actually useful—when engaged properly. Many athletes hurt themselves by *fighting* their fear, telling themselves they *shouldn't* be afraid. That makes the brain turn its attention to . . . well, fighting their fear, instead of dealing with the task at hand. The results are usually disastrous.

Mental health issues can be a nightmare, but when properly understood and managed, they can also become an *advantage*. Given the proper care, some "mental illness" could be seen *not* as an illness, but more like a kind of strength, a divine gift, in need of training. There are levels to mental illness, of course, same as there are levels to physical illness. Yes, it is debilitating if left unchecked, but if properly harnessed, it can be a superpower.

I do not say this lightly. I arrived at this conclusion after my conversations with, among others, Urban Meyer and Mike Gervais. As I talked with Meyer about anxiety, and OCD in particular, he said, "I don't like the term *illness*. Because it's a gift. I'll name you the greatest players, and every one of them has that same trait . . . Think about the greatest athletes. It's not the ones that jump the highest. It's not the ones that run the fastest. It's the one that, when it gets to the edge, they have something God-given that enables them to push right through that."

He explained, saying that when it's the fourth quarter, in a high-pressure situation with the game on the line—that's when ordinary people hit the brakes. "That's common behavior," he said. "Impulsive behavior is to back off. The compulsive, obsessive, high-end, achieving people, those are the ones that keep pushing harder. So I don't think it's an illness. I think you have to be aware of [it] if you have that trait, and how to manage it. But look at it not as an illness, but as a blessing that you somehow have to keep ahold of."

He rattled off the names of one great coach after another, names any sports fan would recognize. "They all share the same quality," Meyer said, "and that's the obsession to be great, and to have a great team. And I don't look at that as a negative. Does that always come with things you have to keep control of? Absolutely."

Apply this idea to a disorder that seems more readily accepted: ADHD (attention deficit hyperactivity disorder). Writer and psychiatrist Dr. Dale Archer, in a July 2014 column for *Forbes*, names a Hall of Fame list of athletes diagnosed with ADHD: Michael Jordan, Michael Phelps, Terry Bradshaw, Pete Rose, Bruce Jenner, Andrés Torres, Cammi Granato. "The list goes on," Archer writes. "This begs the question: is there something about the trait that lends itself to athletic greatness?"

In September 2016, Simone Biles, who won four gold medals at the Rio Summer Olympics, went public with her struggles with ADHD, saying, "I have ADHD and I have taken medicine for it since I was a kid."

Archer, in his column, points out that statistics show that among Major League Baseball players, ADHD is twice as common in the general adult population (9 percent, against 4.4 percent for ages fourteen to forty-four). He also writes, "Many sports psychologists extrapolating from this contend the percentage could be as high as 20 percent among the general pro-athlete population."

Archer goes on to make a compelling argument that can be summed up with this line from his column, based on his review of various scientific findings: "There are many strengths linked to ADHD which, leveraged properly, can lead to success in multiple areas of life."

Among these strengths that would benefit athletes in particular, Archer lists: "the ability to multitask, the propensity to thrive in situations of chaos, creativity, non-linear thinking, an adventurous spirit, resilience, high energy, risk taking, calm under pressure, and the capacity for hyper focus in something that fascinates you."

And, he adds, "I'm not saying it's all good—the problems associated with ADHD are well known—I'm just saying that in our rush to diagnose, we are ignoring that fact that there are indeed positives."

I love all of this, so to check myself, I call Dr. Michael Gervais and ask for his take. He agrees: "Anyone who is world leading, world changing—they are relatively extreme in their dedication, in their ability to go the distance in whatever it is they are pursuing. And by definition, that is rare. And so I don't know if there's a mental illness that would capture the extreme dedication that people have, who are world leading, world changing, but there is, for some people, just the right amount of obsessive-compulsive tendencies, the right amount of anxiousness, the right amount of narcissism, that helps people pursue, to the end of their efforts, the nuances of mastery."

This Stuff, the merging of deep, emerging science and cutting-edge tech, is showing athletes the world in their heads like never before, and helping them push through these fears of their mind in order to explore their true power. Oliver Marmol says, "It's almost the same progression we're seeing with weight lifting and eating, as far as people tapping into the best ways to improve themselves and gain an edge. And as far as what we eat and put into our bodies, everybody is very cautious of that side of improvement when it comes to peak performance. Especially at the highest level, these elite guys are just very conscious of that. So now, looking to how to improve from the neck up—what's possible?"

Someone who learns how to manage what plagues their mind could end up, in fact, doing something "crazy" that ends up being extraordinary—like Felix Baumgartner defeating his fear in order to, with the whole world watching, safely jump from space.

Chapter 6

New Ways to See Old Stuff

Over the years, for better or worse, sports have been rife with various methods of getting one's head in the game, even if that's not how athletes thought of it. And these methods range from quirky to mystical to frightening to damaging to outright bizarre. Sex, superstition, religion, meditation, visualization, self-talk, and the like—many athletes have long sworn by one or the other, while some might swear off all of them entirely.

All of This Stuff throws into sharp perspective our need for getting the mind right—so what does modern science show us about the ways we've already been using to get our minds right? In short: it's showing us how powerful some of it is, both for good, and for bad.

And where that power comes from is how these things drive the production of *neurotransmitters* in the brain. *Neurotransmitter* is basically a fancy word for "brain drug," with neurotransmitters acting in our brain sort of like fuel in a car. Our brain is constantly producing dozens of neurotransmitters, and when we don't need them anymore, the brain soaks up the excess using *reuptakes* so they can be recycled. And in a sense, we are all addicts to these drugs in our brains. The food we eat, drugs we take or don't take, exercise, and so on, and even thoughts and behaviors all deploy various neurotransmitters. To put it one way, our lives are driven by a million little addictions.

And when, say, Russell Wilson has gone automatic—when one "gets into flow"—there's a certain blend that soaks the brain: dopamine, norepinephrine, endorphins, anandamide, and serotonin.

Dopamine shows up when our neocortex successfully predicts the future, such as when we anticipate a threat and avoid it or defeat it. Dopamine makes us feel *good,* making us want to do *more* of whatever it was that made us feel good in the first place. Dopamine also helps us focus and ignore things that don't matter in the moment, and is why going automatic snowballs upon itself. (What sets this dopamine off changes as an athlete becomes better and better, too: one of the starkest differences researchers have found between people who simply play sports for fun—the "hobbyist"—and those who play for a living, or at least are trying to—the "elite"—is that simply *playing* is enough for the hobbyist brain to earn some dopamine, but the elite only get true rewards after experiencing success.)

Norepinephrine is adrenaline, waking the brain up and focusing it, streamlining neuron communication, and affecting our emotional control—kicking us into high gear, making our heart beat faster and our muscles tense and our lungs pump harder.

Endorphins are basically brain-made heroin. They block pain and produce pleasure, like morphine—except they're a hundred times more powerful when produced naturally in the body.

Anandamide is named after the Sanskrit word *ananda,* which means "joy" and "bliss." One of the main things anandamide does is help block out fear, in part by activating *cannabinoid receptors* in the brain.

Finally, *serotonin* helps us cope when things go wrong, and helps keep us calm under pressure. A healthy brain gets dosed with serotonin at the end of an event, whether everything ended up good or bad. When Wilson went from robot to bawling human after that comeback, that's likely because a wave of serotonin was hitting his brain.

Now that you know a bit about what's going on in the brain, let's look at some of the old methods athletes have used to get their minds right, and what science says about them.

SEX

I hate to be the one to break it to you, but *Rocky* lied to us. Specifically, Rocky's trainer, Mick. As he's training Rocky, the punchy southpaw everyman from Philadelphia who nobody thinks has a chance against Apollo Creed/Muhammad Ali, Mick tells him that, under no circumstances, should he have sex: *"Women weaken legs!"*

Good news: Mick—RIP—was wrong.

Or, he might have been wrong. It's complicated, and a difficult thing for science to nail down, and there's not exactly a ton of research out there on the topic. A few studies, most of them with a fairly minimal number of participants.

This has been a hot topic of discussion since the ancient Olympics—Plato himself had something to say on the matter, telling the athletes to save their energy by avoiding sex before competition. However, Pliny the Elder, in 77 A.D., said, "Athletes when sluggish are revitalized by lovemaking."

Freddie Roach, who trains the legendary boxer Manny Pacquiao, among others, has said, "Most boxers abstain for a week or more before a bout—I ask my guys for ten days."

Mike Tyson once said, "I always read that the great fighters never had sex before fights, and I was a young kid, and I wanted to be the youngest heavyweight champion in the world, so I restrained myself from sex for around five years."

Beyond boxing, former top-ranked five-thousand-meter runner Marty Liquori once said, "Sex makes you happy, and happy people don't run a 3:47 mile."

The popular (if not unscientific) belief was that having sex decreased a man's testosterone, thus making him less motivated, less aggressive, less inclined to play hard.

Recent research, however, has found that sex may *increase* a man's level of testosterone—and it's been found that if a man is having regular sex, he'll actually have higher baseline levels of testosterone.

A recent study by Adam & Eve, an erotic goods company, in collaboration with athletic performance coach Dr. Mike Young found that, essentially, as Young puts it, "When it comes to sexual activity and athletic performance it really is a case where an individual's perception is the same as their reality. If they feel like participating in a sexual activity will improve their athletic performance, then it more than likely will."

It's worth taking a closer look, then, at what we *do* know about sex and the brain. First off, sex does fantastic stuff in there. Dopamine, the neurotransmitter that makes us feel good, always shows up. Sex also triggers the release of several other chemicals. There's oxytocin, a painkiller. In fact, the old "not tonight, I have a headache" excuse took a blow after a 2013 German study. In that study, 60 percent of the participants regularly suffered migraines, and 30 percent suffered regular cluster headaches. The study found that the people who had sex reported most, if not all, of their pain going away. Other studies have found that women who orgasm experience an increased pain threshold. Researchers couldn't say for certain why this took place, but they believed it was due to the release of oxytocin.

For an athlete, being able to copulate away aches and pains can be an immense aid to recovery—the less you hurt, the better you rest, and the better you rest, the more quickly you recover.

Sex also shuts down Migsby, our brain's antihero for its major role in vigilance and fear. A break from that is a vacation for the brain, leaving it refreshed and ready for combat.

In addition, sex sends a great deal of blood to the brain. Some studies have even found that regular sex leads to more brain volume—that is, more sex means more brains. Regular sex has also been found to make more neurons grow in the hippocampus, which is important for memory.

On the flip side, some scientific findings indicate that sex is virtually never "just" sex; it is unavoidably emotional. Not only does oxytocin kill pain and make you feel great, but it also generates a vivid imprint on parts of the brain responsible for emotion and memory.

That said, Robert Weiss, the vice president of clinical development at Elements Behavioral Health and an expert in sex addiction, in 2015 wrote for *Psychology Today* that, based on his more than two decades as a psychotherapist specializing in sex and intimacy issues, "At the end of the day, there is no undisputed right or wrong answer when it comes to casual sex and its effects on psychological wellbeing. For some people, it is probably fine, and for others, it is probably not."

SUPERSTITION

Serena Williams wears the same pair of socks for an entire tournament. Michael Jordan wore his old college basketball shorts underneath his NBA shorts, every game. Former college basketball coach Jerry Tarkanian chewed on a towel during games. English football club Birmingham City manager Barry Fry peed in all four corners of his home stadium (to ward off evil spirits). If Jason Giambi, the former MLB slugger, fell into a slump, he'd wear a gold thong during games. Soccer goalkeeper Sergio Goycochea would relieve himself before every penalty kick taken against him.

For no good reason whatsoever, during slow-pitch softball games even to this day, I hit with a certain part of the bat's label facing me, and I have to brush the previous batter's footprints out of the batter's box before I settle in. As a pretentious teenager, I'd tap the plate in the sign of the cross and then tap my chest.

And these are just a few of the countless superstitions held by athletes, perhaps the most superstitious people alive.

It is not really known, yet, what is going on in the brain, physically, when it comes to superstition. Research has found that it likely has to do with Migsby—fear—and other related regions we've already covered. Perhaps the most notable, and concrete, finding scientists have made so far is that people who develop a superstition stay with it, in large part, because rejecting it requires a lot of brainpower that they either don't have or don't feel like using.

Those who do reject superstitions, when their brains were scanned, showed more activity in the *right frontal gyrus,* which is part of the brain linked to *cognitive inhibition*—that is, the part that works to override spontaneous thoughts and emotions.

RELIGION

Plenty of times, growing up, I heard preachers say that good and faithful Christian athletes should be the best in their sports, on account of God's favor and all. A hearty amen to that, I'd say!

As you now know, I demolished that theory. Or maybe God just didn't like me.

Whatever the case, a fascinating correlation between religion and sports has been found: people inclined to sincere belief are also, frequently, better at sports. Dean Hamer, a geneticist who has worked for the National Institutes of Health and the author of *The God Gene,* discovered that when people have a certain variation of a gene called "VMAT2," for whatever reason, they consistently score higher on psychological evaluations that determine how likely they are to hold spiritual and superstitious beliefs. On the athletic side, VMAT2 *also* regulates the flow of dopamine, norepinephrine, and serotonin, and people with that variation get *more* of those neurotransmitters—which makes them better at sports.

In addition, the more that scientists study religion, meditation, and such, the more evidence emerges for how helpful they actually are. "Wisdom of the ancients," Andy Walshe calls it. "The ancient spiritual narrative, when you look at it, was designed very much around human performance. Now, it wasn't called that. It was called *our community survives,* or *we don't fight wars with the neighbors.* It was all called different things. I think religion has clouded a lot of it, and the rhetoric around religion did a disservice. If you shove it down people's throats, as *Do this or you're a bad person going to a bad place,* you're fucking people up. Because that has power. But the concepts of love and dedication and seeking something greater than yourself . . . those were ancient tools."

Walshe makes a good point, and science backs him up: beyond the obvious dangers of fanaticism, an overtly religious upbringing has been found to wreak toxic, severe psychological damage on children. There's even a clinical label: Religious Trauma Syndrome. Dr. Marlene Winell, the psychologist who coined the term, likens RTS to Complex PTSD in her book *Leaving the Fold:* "A psychological injury that results from protracted exposure to prolonged social and/or interpersonal trauma with lack or loss of control, disempowerment, and in the context of either captivity or entrapment, i.e. the lack of a viable escape route for the victim."

One of the major problems with toxic religion is how practitioners twist problems into a gnarled circle of victim blaming. Parents mad at you? Honor them better. Having doubts? *God is testing you, be strong.* Failing at baseball? *Well, so-and-so struggled and prayed and had faith, and became better than ever—are YOU right with God?*

If you're an athlete trying to perform at elite levels with all of that rattling around in your head, forget about it. Migsby will pump full blast, you won't be able to control your heart rate or breathing, Big Fronty will fire on all cylinders, and your brain waves will shoot into a high-beta-dominant pattern. Not only will going automatic become impossible, but you'll also be exhausted.

That said, science has *also* found many ways that people benefit from healthy religion, specifically two of its features that are favorites among athletes: faith and prayer.

FAITH AND PRAYER

Dr. Andrew Newberg at the University of Pennsylvania has spent decades studying the brains of Catholic nuns, Tibetan monks, and the like. His research has found that faith is the "number one best way to exercise your brain . . . Faith is equivalent with hope, optimism, and the belief that a positive future awaits."

This is important because the way we think about *one* thing will often determine the way we later think about something *else.* The brain is a pattern-recognition device. This means that if you're expecting something bad to happen, no matter how good things are going, odds are you'll find something bad to focus on. Ditto for the reverse. Expect good, see good. Our brains only have enough room and energy to hold so much.

Now, obviously, if you're always expecting good things, and then you strike out to lose the game, or crash your car, you're not going to see that as *good,* exactly. But in general, your brain sees more of what it's looking for.

And then there's prayer. Not peacocking disguised as prayer— taking a knee in the end zone after a touchdown, shouting *Thank you, Jesus!* into a microphone, pointing at the sky after home runs and three-pointers—but that still, small voice in our hearts, that conversation with God or Allah or the Flying Spaghetti Monster, and what answers he/she/they might hold. Holding questions in our minds and seeking their answers through thoughtful prayer has a quantifiable effect on our gray matter.

Andrew Newberg has studied how the brains of the devout light up when they pray. He's seen it in Christians, Muslims, Tibetan monks, and more, using a SPECT (*single-photon emission computerized tomography*) scanner, which shows him where the subject's brain is becoming active, and where it is shutting down.

Newberg says that it doesn't matter *what* you focus on, whether it's God or the Bible or math or NASCAR or football. We *might* be hearing the voice of God, *or* we could be *telling* our brains to hear just that. He told NPR, "The more that becomes your reality, the more it becomes written into the neural connections of your brain."

A quick prayer to God during a game can be helpful, but it's a fine line, because too *much* prayer in the middle of performance can trip you up. Intense prayer is intense thought, which gets Big Fronty revved up, which makes your beta waves stronger, too, which drives you further away from automatic, and from the athlete you know you can be.

MEDITATION AND MINDFULNESS

In a way, you could compare prayer to meditation and mindfulness practice, both of which have really come on the scene strong the past few years. *Fortune* magazine reported, in March 2016, how they have become vastly popular on the secular level: "In 2015, the meditation and mindfulness industry raked in nearly $1 billion."

Meditation has long been used by the world's elite athletes—Michael Jordan, Kobe Bryant, and Shaquille O'Neal, for instance, all had the same meditation coach, George Mumford, who taught them about how ancient samurai got into "the zone" and the like, and how to focus less on thoughts like "I've got to make this shot" and to just shoot. "You've trained your nervous system to do it," Mumford once explained to ABC News. "So now your conscious thinking needs to be quiet, and let your body do what it does. Nothing exists but this moment, and what you're doing."

Meditation and mindfulness are, in some ways, different forms of prayer. Or, perhaps more accurately speaking, prayer is another form of meditation. And, to be clear, there are lots of ways to meditate. Transcendental Meditation, Zen meditation, on and on. We don't need to get into all those details here, because there are already plenty of books about them.

Also, meditation and mindfulness like we're talking about here are essentially the same. Remember Russell Wilson and the Seahawks meditating and all that? Dr. Michael Gervais was the one leading them through weekly sessions, and he tells me that while some folks reported that they were doing "guided meditation," he wants to be clear that what he was doing was actually mindfulness training—although he *also* says that the two are virtually the same, at their core.

The important gist is this: whether meditation or mindfulness, the goal for athletes is to become aware of all they are experiencing, and not judge it, stress over it, or have any other sort of unhealthy reaction.

That billion-dollar boom has a lot to do with secular mindfulness and meditation geared around work productivity, but done right, meditation can take people to some profound places. Newberg's colleague Michael Baime, a Tibetan Buddhist whom he studied, meditated an hour a day for forty years. Baime says that, in his meditation zone, he feels at one with the universe and loses all sense of time. "As if the present moment expands to fill all of eternity," he told NPR. "That there has never been anything but this eternal now."

When Newberg watched Baime in his scanner, he saw the parietal lobe go dark, similar to when athletes go automatic. The parietal lobe, remember, processes a lot of sensory input, particularly in order to create a sense of self and orient us in the world. Newberg saw this with monks, Franciscan nuns, chanting Sikhs, and more. In terms of brain activity, Newberg told NPR, "There is no Christian, there is no Jewish, there is no Muslim. It's just all one."

In 2005, Dr. Richard Davidson, a neuroscientist at the University of Wisconsin's W. M. Keck Laboratory for Functional Brain Imaging and Behavior, used EEG scans to study the brains of eight Buddhist monks. These monks had been trained in Tibetan traditions of meditation for around ten thousand to fifty thousand hours over fifteen to forty years. Davidson found that the monks were superb at reaching peak alpha-wave dominance—and, when they focus specifically on, say, an emotion like compassion, they are able to generate bursts of gamma, "the ultimate brain wave," which can reach 100 Hz. (Alpha, remember, is 8 to 12 Hz.) This was, in Davidson's words, "Brain activation on a scale we have never seen before."

This kind of meditative power has taken monks millennia to cultivate, pass down, and master—and so much of what I'm about to cover gets athletes into that same territory.

What's more, early research on even mild meditation for ordinary folks with jobs and crammed schedules shows promise. In 2011, a group of neuroscientists at Harvard studied a group of "normal" people—in other words, not Buddhist monks or Tibetan masters or Pentecostal pastors and such—who followed a guided meditation program for thirty minutes a day. Using MRI, the scientists saw detectable changes in the subjects' brains within two months, trending toward what masters could do.

In a Harvard study published in 2011, neuroscientists found mindfulness rebuilding brains' gray matter.

Neuroscientists at the University of Wisconsin's Laboratory for Affective Neuroscience, back in 2003, performed an eight-week study with forty-one employees from a biotech company. They were split into two groups. A group of twenty-five people received a mindfulness-based stress reduction program; the remaining sixteen did nothing, to serve as a control group. The test group went through quite the meditation boot camp: a class every week, daily one-hour meditation homework, and a seven-hour retreat. After about two months, their results were stunning: not only did their brains physically change, their immune system did, too. The researchers injected the test group with a flu vaccine, drew their blood, ran some tests, and found that they had more flu virus antibodies compared to the control group. Using EEG assessments, the researchers found that the test group subjects' brains were more activated in regions associated with positive emotions and resilience, some of which also coordinate with, you guessed it, the immune system.

Let's take a second to look at the neuroscience of mindfulness and meditation. It's wild: meditation creates such calm because it disconnects you from, well, *you,* by changing how parts of the brain connect.

The *lateral prefrontal cortex* drives rational, logical, balanced thought, and is responsible for managing emotional responses, overriding habits, and the like. This is known as the *assessment center.*

The *medial prefrontal cortex* connects all of your experience to shape your perspective. This is the *me center,* the part of the brain obsessed with *you* and the people around you. It has two sections: the *ventromedial medial prefrontal cortex* (vmPFC) and the *dorsomedial prefrontal cortex* (dmPFC).

The vmPFC processes information related to you and folks you think are like you, and is to blame when you take things too personally and ruminate, which exacerbates anxiety and depression.

The dmPFC processes information about people who are different from you. This part is crucial—it helps you empathize and feel compassion.

Then the insula, which we've covered already, monitors bodily sensations, governs how strongly you respond to things, and also helps with empathy.

Finally, there's Migsby, our infamous little seat of the fear center, freaking us out, sparking our fight-or-flight response.

Dr. Rebecca Gladding, a clinical instructor and attending psychiatrist at UCLA, broke down the physical aspects of this in a February 2013 article for *Psychology Today.* For starters, she wrote, before people start meditating, there are lots of neural connections within the me center, as well as between the me center and the parts of the brain handling bodily sensation—and promoting fear.

This is important because, in other words, when you feel worried, or scared, or feel something like an itch or pain, your brain's more likely to tell you that something's wrong and your safety is in jeopardy—and that's the Me Center handling things. That's why we'll get stuck in looping negative thought about our lives, our mistakes, what people think about us, and so on.

This is all because of a weak connection between the me center and the assessment center.

Make the assessment center stronger and the part of the brain taking everything personally will calm down, and the part that understands others will get way better. According to Gladding, the assessment center works as a brake, slowing the me center down when it gets running too hard.

And yeah, meditation can make the connection between the me center and assessment center stronger, which changes everything.

First, good meditation weakens the link between the me center and the sensory and fear centers, which is typically quite strong at first. When it weakens, you don't automatically connect a brief physical feeling or a brush of fear with something being horribly *wrong*. This is super helpful for people with anxiety. You learn to ignore the stuff that makes you anxious, as the neural links between upsetting sensations and the me center fade away.

And, since your assessment center starts working better, instead of assuming everything is some kind of threat, you get better at taking a beat to recognize what's really going on. The link between the assessment center and the sensory and fear centers gets stronger, and that better helps you to pause, to not just *react*, and to process from a more rational perspective. For instance, when you feel a pain in your leg, you can just let it go instead of . . . oh, I don't know, imagining the horrific infection that's going to get your leg amputated at the kneecap.

On top of all that, meditation helps the *dorsomedial prefrontal cortex*—the good part of the me center, responsible for empathy—by strengthening its links to the part of the brain that handles the body's sensory input. Because of *that,* the part of your brain that interprets other people's thoughts and feelings starts working better, so then you're better at connecting with people and, say, seeing things from their perspective.

The key, Gladding says, is daily practice. If you stop, same as with working out, you'll lose some gains, but if you stay on top of it, when you really need it, your brain will work for you.

Some of This Stuff helps us develop the same abilities as those monks, such as a product called Muse that uses EEG technology to create, as is the company motto, "meditation made easy." Dan Chartier recommended I check it out. Muse is a sleek piece of hardware that wraps around the forehead and settles on your ears, almost like a reverse set of headphones, except it doesn't go on your ears, but behind them. It has five sensors, three on the forehead and two behind the ears.

Before every session, Muse takes a minute to "calibrate" your brain activity to its app, and then you begin. You can do it as long or as short as you want. By default, the app comes with a beach scene and sounds, which get louder the more active your brain becomes and more quiet the calmer your brain gets. When you get really calm, you hear birds chirping. Using an app—also free to download—Muse guides you through meditation and helps you calm your mind. Chartier—who has no stake in Muse—says that he's had patients bring Muse headbands into his office and wear them while he straps them into his medical-grade EEG setup, and Muse is accurate. Not as thorough as his stuff, but what it aims to do, it does well.

However they do it, athletes are getting more into mindfulness every year. Mike Gervais says, "Samurai warriors were deeply attracted to the Zen traditions so they could become more present, so they could adjust to the sword in front of them. And basically, the Zen traditions are teaching mindfulness. Now it's a defining feature of elite athletes."

VISUALIZATION

A close cousin to mindfulness, visualization can mean a few different things, but they all accomplish the same goal: use a mental image to get into the mind-set you want. This is another classic psychological technique popular among athletes. Russell Wilson, for instance, wrote an essay for the *Player's Tribune* describing one of his visualization techniques: a big reset button. Specifically, he references the comeback against Green Bay, writing, "It seemed like everything that could go wrong had gone wrong. Personally, I was having one of my worst games of my career. But after every single throw—whether it was a tipped ball or an incompletion or a touchdown—I'd turn back toward the huddle, close my eyes and think of a table in an empty room. On that table was a big red RESET button, just like in the movies. I'd imagine pressing the button. *Boom*. On to the next one. What's the situation now? How can I make a play?"

There are a million ways to incorporate visualization, and like all of these classic methods, it's well-trod territory in plenty of other books, so we won't go deeper in the weeds here than we need, except to identify some of the practitioners and use this knowledge to examine the science behind the technique.

Jordan Spieth, the 2015 Masters champ and, as of this writing, the number two golfer in the world, openly talks about visualization. TV microphones often catch his caddie giving him visuals to focus on as Spieth lines up his shot.

And maybe the most compelling example of a guy who's gotten a lot out of visualization is Jason Day, the Australian golfer currently ranked number one in the world. He began working with performance coach Jason Goldsmith in early 2013 or so. They devised an intensive fifteen-step process heavy on visualization that enables Day, as he puts it, to achieve *mushin,* Japanese for "mind of no-mindedness." In the zone.

Day's routine begins with two practice swings, during which he feels out his ideal swing while concentrating on his shot. Then he steps back, closes his eyes, and pictures himself standing a few feet in front of himself, about to hit. He sees his swing go back and then through the ball, and then he sees the ball fly away; then he watches where it goes, how it lands, and how it bounces. And, he says, he keeps visualizing until he feels comfortable.

The initial visual takes him just a few seconds. Then he approaches the ball, looking downrange, picking a target. As he steps over the ball to take his position, he keeps his head up and his eyes on the target—say, a tower, or a tree in line with where he wants the ball to go. Then he looks back to the ball while consciously holding on to the image of that target. His "awareness going back out," as he describes it. Then he looks up to the target once more, locking it in his mind, before he will "throw my awareness back to the ball." He waggles the club to loosen up, resets the club behind the ball, and then, *blammo.*

The whole process, from practice swings to blammo, takes maybe ten to fifteen seconds. You might easily never know it was happening.

"The biggest thing," he has said before, "is to aim small, miss small. It's like shooting at a target. You don't shoot at the whole target, especially if you have a gun, or a bow and arrow. You try to hit that little center piece."

Day and Goldsmith have been talking about all of this at least since 2014. Goldsmith explained to Golf.com, "The reason why golf is so difficult is because you're starting the action—everything is still, so your intellect wants to be involved. Your mind wants to be in control, but the golf swing has to be done on a subconscious level. It's impossible to think about the thousands of muscles and tendons and ligaments that have to fire in a perfect sequence in a fraction of a second. Yet even the best players in the world get stuck in a pattern of trying to consciously make the perfect swing. It doesn't work."

Day's visualization routine developed over time as he and Goldsmith analyzed data generated by a brain-reading sweatproof headband called FocusBand, a rare EEG product that seems to work out in the field. I say rare because, remember, the slightest movement or flexing of muscles in the face and scalp causes inaccurate spikes in EEG readings—a clenched jaw, an eyeblink, even rolling your eyes.

That said, FocusBand purportedly works, at least with a "still" sport like golf.

After he turned pro in 2006 at age eighteen, Jason Day's career was solid going into 2012, finishing second twice in major tournaments and winning three smaller professional tournaments, but no majors. In 2012, Goldsmith was part of a team in Australia led by businessman Henry Boulton and his father, Graham, who developed FocusBand to help golfers know when they are calm enough to take a swing.

That is, when they are *mushin*. Day loved it.

This works by way of three brain sensors woven into the fabric, located on the forehead, the temple, and behind the ear. When you use a computer or smartphone, you're shown an avatar that provides several different means of real-time feedback, including facial tension, anxiety, focus, "left brain"—by which they mean whether you are thinking too much—and "right brain," which is when, they say, you have achieved *mushin*.

Skeptical when I first heard all of this, I called Chartier and asked him about it. He'd never heard of FocusBand, and I told him that I wasn't too sure about that whole left-brain/right-brain deal. He said there's actually science to back that up.

We've all heard of left-brain/right-brain personalities—supposedly if people are more analytical and logical and all that, they are left-brain dominant, and right-brain dominant if they're more artsy and intuitive and the like. This is not necessarily true on a scientific level, although—and I might oversimplify this—basically the left hemisphere of the brain is responsible for thinking things through—strategizing a game plan—while the right brain handles intuition and instinct and the like—feeling out the best plays in specific situations. Apparently, a bottleneck effect can occur as the brain processes information and input, and if you're overthinking—say, when you're trying to hit a golf ball—then that cramps away the space your instincts need to help you physically perform.

That's what FocusBand purportedly helps you clarify.

Day's pursuit of *mushin* and his use of the FocusBand, like so much other mental-work stuff throughout the history of sports, drew ridicule. A golf writer covering the Masters for Grantland in April 2013 wrote that Day's pursuit of *mushin* and his FocusBand sounded "like an absurd invention from a bad sci-fi show or the brainchild of a 19th-century snake oil salesman."

Three years after that, however, in August 2016, Day has fifteen professional wins, including the 2015 PGA Championship—his first major—and he is the number-one-ranked golfer in the world.

MIRRORING

Another aspect of what makes visualization so effective is a phenomenon that I call "mirroring." (No idea if someone else used that term before me; sorry if you have, but I couldn't find you on the Google.) Back in my college days, before I knew about any of this, I experienced mirroring on an intense level with no clue what was going on. If I'd had any idea, I would've used it all the time, and I'd be a millionaire all-star World Series MVP by now. Okay, maybe not, but I would have at least, you know, not sucked.

Mirroring occurs when athletes watch someone else playing their sport: their brain processes *watching* as though they are actually *doing* what they see.

Before one game my junior year of college, during batting practice, the other team was launching balls out of the park. Just bomb, bomb, bomb. That was their thing. Ridiculous, and yeah, fun to watch.

Now, my team, on the other hand—our BP didn't look quite so impressive. Our coach had a specific routine we had to follow. I don't remember what it was exactly—something like hit a ball opposite field, do a hit-and-run, two-strike swings, and the like. And we weren't hitting great that day. It was freezing cold—our seasons started on February 1 every year, which was miserable—and guys were having a rough time.

I noticed the other team in their dugout, most of them watching us and laughing. I was already frustrated with baseball, so when it was my turn to hit, I stepped into the box angry. Since I was a head case, *angry* normally meant "tense" and "play like crap," but that day, for some reason, I was different. Stupid as this sounds now, that batting practice is one of my favorite college baseball memories. Ordinarily, I was a righteous follower of Coach's rules. But that day, I said to hell with them and swung away.

In my anger, I felt something so rare back then. I felt free.

And I hit the crap out of the ball.

I wasn't thinking about the other team laughing. I wasn't thinking about proving my coach or my teammates or anyone else wrong. I was just mad—and I kept seeing the other team swinging free and for power. Like how I once could.

Opposite-field swing, hit-and-run swing, two-strike swing—I hit almost every pitch out of the park, and many of them way out, over the scoreboard, high into pine trees beyond the fence. The field went quiet. When I stepped out of the box, one of my team-mates said, "Damn, Sneed, what got into you?"

Same thing happened before the game I hit my first home run. I'd been watching a rerun of a Home Run Derby before a game that, for whatever reason, Coach put me in the starting lineup for. I felt pretty good, even though it was another miserable, cold day. I got hits my first three at-bats—single, double, triple. And then, my last at-bat, I hit my first college home run. Miracle of miracles, I wound up in the starting lineup for the *next* game, too. And the weirdest thing happened: I was so high on confidence that I could even throw the ball back to the pitcher.

Now that I write this out, I want to go back and shake Past Brandon and tell him that that's probably what Coach was wait-ing for all along. To get mad, to get anything, to make myself stop thinking so much. To quote every former athlete ever, if only I'd known then what I know now—because it all faded within a couple games, and back to the bench I went.

Anyway, here's the science: some of our neurons are called "mirror neurons." They send signals through the brain that mir-ror activity we witness. In a way, they translate what you *see* as though you are actually *doing* it your brain. They are, in part, why it's so hard to stay calm when someone else is upset with you, for example. They're partly why television and movies are so popular (not to mention porn). They play a role in riots—massive groupthink taking over, everyone seeing everyone around them acting a certain way registering in their brain as *them* acting that way, too, and eventually, their bodies follow their brains.

And they are why we love watching sports.

This can go so far, with practice, that even simply *thinking* about doing something registers in your brain as if you are actually doing it. I found some studies on people shooting free throws. In one study, one group shoots free throws, another group simply visualizes shooting them, and another group doesn't practice at all. The group that practiced improved, the group that didn't practice at all, obviously, didn't improve—but the group that visualized shooting improved as much as the group that actually practiced.

SELF-TALK

Upon introducing an exercise in Nike's new app, Nike Football Pro Genius, Joe Hart, the goalkeeper for Manchester City and the England national team, says, "Our thoughts . . . have a huge impact on how we feel. If you can learn how to think before a game, you can influence your performance on the pitch. Self-talk is a technique that positively manages your inner voice. It only takes a few minutes and helps you prepare for the ninety ahead. Let any negative thoughts go, and replace them with the positive 'I can' or 'I will' statements. Like, 'I can stop anything,' or, 'I will dominate my area.'"

Self-talk combines with visualization to manage your thoughts. In other words, where visualization is *seeing* something in order to generate a mental state you want, self-talk is consciously thinking things to yourself—or even saying them out loud—to do the same. Hart says he focuses on a great game he's played before. For his pregame routine, he closes his eyes for a few minutes in the locker room and remembers March 17, 2015, when Manchester City faced Barcelona in the UEFA Champions League tournament—Hart against Lionel Messi and the rest of "the world's most feared attack."

Other than an Ivan Rakitić goal—described by broadcasters as "sumptuous"—midway through the first half, Hart allowed nothing. Blond, blue-eyed, tall, and fantastic, he played like a god that day, leaving even Messi in awe. "He was saving every ball," Messi said after the game. "He even saved some balls with his chest. Really top-notch."

"Now," Hart says, "I mentally replay every save I made. I draw on the positive feelings they gave me at the time. My routine fills me with the belief that I will play at my best. It makes me realize that the only person who can beat me is me."

Hart says all of this introducing that new app, but I mention it here because what Hart is saying is based in solid psychology and neuroscience.

For instance, if you constantly tell yourself "Don't get out, don't miss this free throw, don't fumble this ball, don't doof this move," then what you are really doing is telling your brain "Get out. Miss this shot. Fumble. Doof." (When I constantly thought, *Don't throw the ball away* . . . well, away the ball was thrown.)

Reason: when you do this, the brain translates the words like *no* and *not* as . . . nothing. They don't register.

Since your brain competes with itself for resources, it can be pretty well conditioned to focus on either positive or negative things in life. This sounds hokey, but science bears it out: the more someone complains, the more they'll find reasons to complain, and the more someone finds something to be happy about, the more they'll find things *to* be happy about.

Another example: simply *thinking I'm so angry right now* or *I'm so scared* and the like only makes your brain double down on that emotion. When your brain hears "I am," whatever follows registers as a statement about your very *identity*, compelling your brain to begin taking steps to make it permanent. Your brain translates emotion—"I am angry"—to "being angry is who I am."

This activates our fight-or-flight response and makes us feel more threatened, which only makes the problem worse.

Researchers have found ways around this, thank goodness: shift *I* am *this way* to *I* feel *this way.* This changes blood flow in the brain, moving it away from Migsby and other regions associated with fight-or-flight, and toward the Big Fronty, which handles critical thinking, empathy, and problem solving.

Some experts take this a step further, beyond even, say, *I* feel *angry* to *I* am doing *anger.* This works in the brain by creating an illusion of control over the emotion. This is useful because the mind's illusions often create the brain's reality.

And not just for emotions. Science has found the mind to be capable of literally healing us—or making us sick.

PLACEBO

Like all of us, I'd heard of the placebo effect, but I had no idea just how powerful it can be.

Scott Schafer, a Colorado University–Boulder grad student in 2015 working for Associate Professor Tor Wager's Cognitive and Affective Neuroscience Lab in the department of psychology and neuroscience, published a remarkable study that May. Over four sessions, he gave subjects a placebo that he told them eliminated pain, and they said it worked—and then, when he *told* them it was a placebo, then ran more tests, the placebo *still* worked.

The same concept has been applied to a variety of different ailments. For example, in a study published in January 2010, gastroenterologists at the Wake Forest University School of Medicine found that a placebo caused remission in patients with Crohn's disease.

On the flip side, there's a lesser-known phenomenon called the "nocebo effect." Dr. Lissa Rankin, author of *Mind Over Medicine*, writes about study subjects who have been given placebo pills, warned about their potential side effects—which didn't actually exist—and then became sick. She writes, "Patients given nothing but saline who thought it was chemotherapy actually threw up and lost their hair!"

In Australia, aboriginal tribes believe that if a medicine man points a bone at someone who committed a crime, that person will die; sometimes, this actually happens. (When it doesn't, it's because the bone-pointing was done incorrectly.) Belief in such voodoo is still common and strong enough that hospital staff will go beyond basic medicine to provide "counter-magic," the only "treatment" that can "cure" the afflicted.

In March 2006, a study of 1,800 surgery patients conducted by a large group of researchers from Harvard Medical School, Beth Israel Medical Center, the Benson-Henry Institute for Mind Body Medicine, Integris Baptist Medical Center in Oklahoma City, the Mayo Clinic, and the Washington Hospital Center in D.C. found that surgery patients who knew that people were praying for them ended up faring *worse* than patients who were told nobody was praying for them, or patients who were told that people might or might not be praying for them.

Then there's this stunning example of the nocebo effect: a study at the Oxford Centre for Functional MRI of the Brain in 2011, led by professor of anaesthetic science Irene Tracey, while studying the efficacy of an opioid drug, found that something that *should* be effective can be rendered useless after a subject is told it *won't* work. That's right: even though something is scientifically proven to help people—such as a pill—if people decide it's not going to work, sometimes it won't.

Ditto for This Stuff. If athletes go into any of this cynical, it might not help them.

Then there is simply this power of awareness. (Back to that word again.) I found dozens of breathtaking stories while researching all of this that don't fit the scope of this book, but there is one I can't stop thinking about. In 2007, Harvard psychologist Ellen Langer studied maids with body fat, waist-hip ratios, blood pressure, weight, and BMIs all in the unhealthy ranges seen in people who don't get enough exercise—even though the maids were on their feet and moving all day, and usually while hauling around those heavy carts. Their job was tailor-made for fitness. In fact, the maids technically got *more* exercise than the U.S. surgeon general's basic recommendations. And yet they were far from fit.

Langer split eighty-four maids into two groups. She didn't tell one group anything. She told the other group how many calories they were actually burning, and how they were getting more than enough exercise. That's it.

A month later, the informed group lost weight, slimmed down, and saw a 10 percent drop in blood pressure.

Simply by being told they should get better, they got better.

Getting athletes to understand the power of their minds has traditionally meant talking it out. And that's only if the athlete is open to talking. Even now that remains difficult, but the only way to get the mind right is to have these conversations.

That's where This Stuff is changing things, especially the new, cutting-edge tech. Nothing starts a conversation quite like showing someone their brain on a screen, or, as we're about to see, using a scientifically engineered system to thrust them into a meditative state, or putting them in a virtual-reality simulation where they feel safer simply saying, "Yeah, this is hard for me."

Oliver Marmol, the minor league baseball coach, says that athletes today are having conversations the likes of which were nonexistent among athletes even a single generation ago. "The generation coming up is very in tune with how to use technology to improve things," he says. "The more tech comes out, and the more they use it, the more open they are to talking about how they feel when they're using it. The language they use starts to re-volve around, *this is how I'm processing this at this time . . .* Now that we're able to load their systems with tech out there, and have them verbalize it in a training setting where it's controlled, it's safe, there's no consequences, they become familiar with that, and carry it out to their game."

This sets up a brave new world full of growing pains and stag-gering potential, the Wild West of training all over again. "On the physical side, we could work out until the cows come home, and we have certain limitations physically," Marmol says. "At some point, genetically, you're just going to tap out. But from the neuro side, there's just endless amounts of gains there that elite athletes even at the highest level aren't even tapping into yet."

In other words, here comes the revolution.

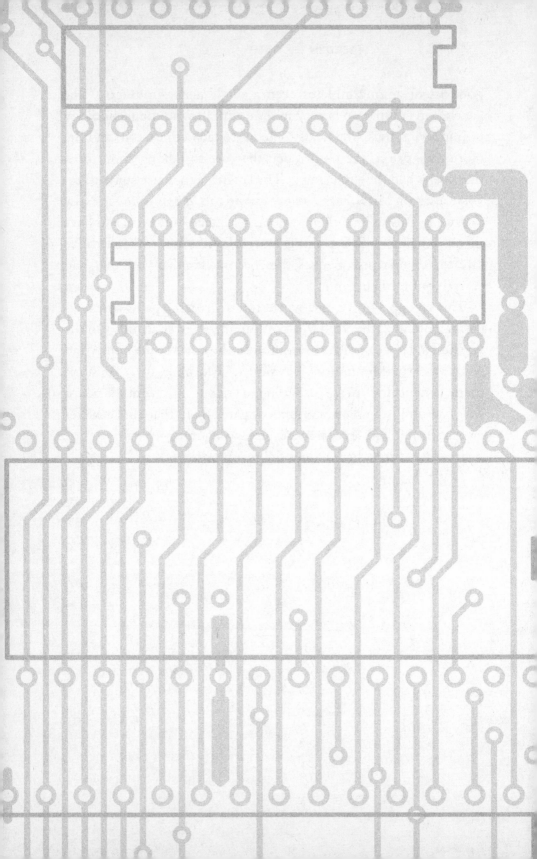

PART TWO

THE BODY

The heart has reasons that reason cannot know.

—Blaise Pascal

Chapter 7

The Power of a Proper Breath

Aristotle believed that the seat of human thought and consciousness was not in the brain but in the heart.

Believe it or not, he wasn't that far off. Maybe one of the most awe-inspiring things I've learned is that for as many millions of signals as the brain sends to our heart, the heart sends *double* that number to the brain.

Why this is and what it means remains a mystery, but the implication is clear: the brain isn't as in control as it seems. The heart does a lot of telling the brain what to do. There is a *sinoatrial node* that links with the *vagus nerve* (pronounced "VAY-gis") to connect the heart to the limbic part of the brain—that's the reactive part, which generates our more animal-like basic instincts and desires.

This is freaky, because it feels like something we can't control. But we can.

That's why I'm in Montreal in January 2016, meeting with Dr. Pierre Beauchamp. He knows how.

We meet at a café near the University of Montreal on the Chemin de la Côte-des-Neiges. He wears glasses and has white hair, and he orders us cappuccinos. Through his sports consultation company, Mindroom, Beauchamp works with elite athletes the world over, including direct work with some of Canada's premier Olympians, and consults with great teams and athletes, such as A.C. Milan and the Ferrari F1 auto racing team. I'm here because he offered to show me all things Mindroom.

But first, regarding my general research, he asks, "What's been most helpful to you so far?"

I jabber away about EEG training—and immediately it's clear that Beauchamp doesn't share my enthusiasm. "EEG hasn't been used in Olympic sport in the way you're describing," he says. His concern is the same as most EEG skeptics: "There's not enough proof yet that it actually works. So you have to be careful with that." That said, Beauchamp adds, "Now, I've done EEG with Olympic athletes, and I've got some other colleagues who have done EEG with Olympic athletes—but we don't say what we're doing, because the people inside sports science might shoot [us]."

Beauchamp says that he used to be a hockey player, and then a hockey coach, and, he says, "If I walk into a pro hockey locker room, and say, 'I'm going to do EEG,' they're going to throw me out. 'You're not attaching any wires to my players' brains!'"

Make no mistake, I'm here because Beauchamp believes in training the brain—but in a different way, one that I think Aristotle would love: managing the mind by addressing the brain *first* is good and helpful in some ways, but Beauchamp calls that "a top-down method" that he doesn't believe always works. His own methods, also based in deep science, are what he calls "the bottom-up approach."

That is, to master the mind, first master the body.

Specifically, master the heart.

Many years ago, Beauchamp went to a baseball game. As he watched the pregame batting practice, he was captivated by a Seattle rookie with a sweet swing, hitting the ball for miles. Nothing unusual about that in and of itself—big leaguers always mash in BP. But as the game started, Beauchamp kept watching him, because the kid had a rare demeanor, an easy, almost preternatural coolness and focus.

"I was so impressed with him as an individual," Beauchamp says now, a far-off look in his eye. "His ability in the warm-up to be focused, and then his ability, for nine innings, to be completely focused, and to manage everything that was going on around him—already, so young. When athletes are stressed or not focused, they're looking in the stands, they're looking at the skirts, just too much trash talking with the guys. But he was getting centered. Feeling his environment. Totally in control. He wasn't overdoing it. He was just in the moment. And the way he ripped the ball—I can't remember how many hits he got, but he *hit* the ball, and I think he got a homer. I was just so impressed at his overall ability, handling all that was going on—knowing that he was that young, a rookie. And I said to myself then, *He is going to be Hall of Fame material one day.*"

Unbeknownst to Beauchamp, that kid had indeed been voted into the Hall of Fame just the week before we met—and by a record margin at that, with 99.32 percent of the votes, breaking the previous record of 98.84 percent held by Tom Seaver. That kid was *the* Kid, Ken Griffey Jr.

To put it one way, Beauchamp's mission is to help athletes tap into their inner Ken Griffey Jr. He does it by teaching them the secrets of the athletic body, which he knows the way computer engineers know motherboards. "René Descartes thought the brain and the body were separate," Beauchamp tells me. "We've come a long way since. Now we know that it's bidirectional. It works both ways. There's a two-way channel. There is the brain to the heart, and the heart to the brain. And what that does is, it controls your nervous system."

A few hours after Beauchamp and I meet at the café, we're on the second floor of an office building across the street, sitting in a small room that is empty except for a table and a couple of chairs. (They're remodeling.) Beauchamp opens a big gray briefcase full of medical equipment. Monitors, sensors, that sort of stuff. He pulls out a laptop, sets it on the table, and opens a program called BioGraph Infiniti. Then he puts an infrared sensor on my finger and straps a black elastic belt with some sort of sensor on it around my stomach.

The finger sensor measures my heart rate. The stomach belt, my breathing.

For fifteen minutes, he puts me through a series of breathing exercises that make me follow a pacer on the computer. "In through the nose, and with your belly," Beauchamp says. "And then out, with pursed lips. Always use your belly. Not your thorax." He tells me that the idea here is, "Doing effortless breathing. You're breathing smoothly, rhythmically, in an effortless way."

He coaches me from eight breaths per minute down to five. When we finish, he explains that this is all to test my *heart rate variability* in order to find my *resonance frequency*. I just assumed my heartbeat's rhythm was fairly steady, but his tech shows me that no, much like my dancing, my heart's rhythm is all over the place. The resonance frequency is when my heartbeat is steadiest. "Every athlete has a resonance frequency that's individual," Beauchamp says. The tests give his software some data, and the software will use that data to generate what he calls the HRV Report. "This is software I developed for sport," he says, studying the data on the screen. "And it says your best breathing rate is seven-point-oh. Seven breaths per minute."

The program arrives at that conclusion by analyzing when I am producing my strongest breaths combined with the steadiest beating of my heart. Beauchamp says, "That's when you achieve *homeostasis.*"

Homeostasis is the perfect balance between the sympathetic and parasympathetic nervous systems. Our sympathetic system is responsible for arousal. Too much sympathetic activation, and an athlete is too fired up—or too nervous. Fight-or-flight mode, overactivated.

Parasympathetic is the inverse. Parasympathetic calms you down. Too much of this, and an athlete is going to be sluggish, unmotivated, disengaged.

Homeostasis puts us right in the middle, perfectly alert and aware and active, but also perfectly calm. That's where athletes want to be in order to perform their best. And, according to Beauchamp, they can reach homeostasis by finding their perfect breathing rate—which, for me, is apparently seven breaths per minute.

Also, a brief aside about the parasympathetic system: it is captained by the vagus nerve, which is a long nerve strand that, to oversimplify, runs all the way from our brain down through our internal organs. Its name comes from the fact that it "wanders" vagabond-style through the body. The vagus nerve has an array of responsibilities, too—managing inflammation, helping make memories, telling you to breathe, and, among others, helping manage your heart rate.

It is this nerve that sends electrical impulses to the aforementioned sinoatrial node, which releases *acetylcholine,* a critical neurotransmitter for performance. Acetylcholine is crucial for muscle function, and it works as a *neuromodulator,* altering the way other brain structures process information. That is, when other neurotransmitters send information, in *cholinergic areas* of the brain, acetylcholine manages the flow of that information, and many such areas play an important role in keeping us alert, focused, and motivated.

When Beauchamp trains athletes to manage their heart-rate variability, he is essentially training them to use their breathing, which directly affects the heart, to take control of their vagus nerve.

Beauchamp attaches sensors to two more of my fingers. These, he says, measure my *skin conductance.* Our skin gives off electricity, apparently. The sensors measure how much. "Skin conductance is a good measure of how stressed you are," he says. The calmer you are, he explains, the more your skin temperature rises, and the lower your skin conductance falls. "This is a lie detector," he says. Same thing cops use. "Well, kind of. This is a lot more sensitive than what the cops have."

He tells me to exhale every 3.3 seconds and inhale every 5.2, thus taking a full breath every 8.5 seconds, which puts me almost dead-on seven breaths per minute. In through the nose, out through pursed lips, always using the belly.

As I do this, he studies his laptop screen and nods. We train for about fifteen minutes and he teaches me how to achieve homeostasis on my own. The process takes some work, and a lot of adjusting and looking at jagged lines on a computer screen and trying to smooth them out—but by the end, I'm getting the hang of it, and I'm feeling good and calm, and Beauchamp is pleased. "You are now controlling your nervous system with your breathing," he says, with a smile that seems to add, *And without plugging anything onto your skull.*

He says that now that I know my resonance frequency, I can train myself with any bio-breathing app, and that after two to three weeks, breathing at that frequency should become subconscious.

"Now," he says, "let's go do a NeuroTracker session."

We go back downstairs and into a room with half the lights turned off. There's a big 3-D flat screen on the wall, hooked to a computer. I sit on a stool about ten feet from the TV and put on 3-D goggles. NeuroTracker is, essentially, a computer game designed to measure and train cognitive processing. It was created in the University of Montreal's cognitive research lab a few years ago.

Beauchamp turns on the computer and fires up NeuroTracker. Eight yellow balls appear on-screen, four highlighted orange. Then the highlights disappear and the balls start flying around. Basically, it's a high-tech shell game on steroids, driven by an algorithm that makes the balls move faster or slower depending on how well you perform. The balls fly around in 3-D for eight seconds, and then I have to identify which ones were highlighted in the beginning. Twenty rounds equal one session.

Beauchamp says how well someone does at NeuroTracker, in part, provides a "neurocognitive measure" of their focusing and processing skills. When someone is stressed, their Migsby kicks into gear, and their body and brain produce *cortisol*, "the stress hormone." Long-term exposure to cortisol can *shrink* the hippocampus—which forms new memories—and the prefrontal cortex, thus reducing one's ability to focus and process.

A few hours ago, after we met at the café, I did my first session, and I scored a 1.88. Although the scoring is a bit confusing, Beauchamp told me that 1.88 was my "speed threshold," or the level of speed, on average, at which I was able to correctly identify all four highlighted balls. By comparison, well-trained elite athletes can score around 4.0 or even higher—so I was terrible, though Beauchamp insisted that my score was pretty good for a first-timer.

My second session about half an hour ago went even worse. It took place after about two hours of interviewing Beauchamp, who walked me through all kinds of deep science—and I scored 0.9.

"Before," Beauchamp had said, "you were primed. We'd just

had lunch. And you came in and did a 1.88. Then we had lectures, right? And now it's three thirty, when most people are normally fatigued, a low point in your circadian rhythm. And you've been listening for a long time, and taking in a lot of information. The brain is tired now. We tested you. And you were half of what you were two hours ago."

"Coffee, man!" I said. "I needed my coffee."

"You weren't allowed, though. That's a performance-enhancing stimulant." He smiled like a master.

"So this is basically what you expected."

"Yes. And my point is, we must think of all the athletes showing up at the clubhouse for a game. They're all in different states of readiness. What kind of warm-ups are they doing to get them ready? And are they peaking at the start of the game? And can they maintain it for, say, nine innings? That's not an easy thing to do."

I laughed. "So you know what you're doing here."

He grinned. "Now you're getting it. You cognitively cannot do any more training from the neck up, from the head down. Would you agree?"

"Yeah," I said. "That was rough. I did not enjoy it."

After this, Beauchamp had taken me back to the office, hooked me up, and taught me about resonance frequencies and homeostasis.

Now he says we're going to use what he taught me to make me good at NeuroTracker again. Not too jacked up, not too chilled out.

At first, I keep struggling, same as during my second session. Beauchamp pauses the game and talks me through the breathing. "You're learning here," he says. "When you lose focus, how do you get it back? A good place to get it back is the breathing. To get back in the game, just take a breath."

The idea behind Beauchamp's approach is not to train your brain to stay in a certain zone, but rather to train yourself to control your body in a way that, say, focuses your brain and keeps it primed to perform.

When the session ends, I've done well, scoring a 1.68, and that's only because I blinked on the last two turns. I should have scored higher than 2.0. "You screwed me up!" Beauchamp says with a grin. "I was about to make myself look so good!" We laugh and Beauchamp adds, "But the numbers aren't really important. It's the process."

One of the biggest problems with typical coaches right now, he says, is that even if they try to address mental conditioning, they start with immediately trying to change the athlete's thinking. "They forget about the underlying stuff," Beauchamp says. "It may work in the moment, but if you want long-lasting change, you need a way for the athlete, on a daily basis, to be able to be in control."

That, he says, is one of the important differences between head-down and bottom-up approaches to the mind. Head-down can only be used outside of a game—you can't take EEG onto the field with you. Bottom-up, however, teaches athletes techniques they can use and feel out right in the middle of competition. "Athletes with tens or hundreds of thousands of people watching, clapping, yelling—we need to know that we can help the athlete cope with that environment," Beauchamp says.

And here, too, is a crucial point: "We're not asking them to perform like Superman. We just want them to perform optimally. Because under high stress, if you try to perform like Superman, you're doing something wrong."

That said, Beauchamp knows that keeping the mind relaxed yet focused for extended periods of time is hard and a skill almost everyone takes for granted. Thus, Mindroom.

A few years ago, a local newspaper writer described Beauchamp as a psychologist and compared Mindroom to the horrifying treatment the villain gets in Stanley Kubrick's *A Clockwork Orange*.

And because of articles like that, Beauchamp now avoids giving interviews. "That guy screwed me," he says.

So before I get into anything else, let's be clear on what both Mindroom and Beauchamp are and what they are not. This will give us a better understanding of the variations in the different ways people can approach training in and with This Stuff.

First, Beauchamp is a sports *scientist*. He's not being pedantic by spelling this out for me, like a professor who insists on a student calling him "Doctor." No, labels—and mislabelings—are a real problem in the worlds of sports science and psychology, as many claim to be sports psychologists who, in fact, are not. "Sports psychology is very hot," Beauchamp says. After the newspaper guy screwed him, Beauchamp says, "I was up against the order of psychologists. And I said, 'Listen, I totally agree with you guys. Here's my card. This is what I gave him.' But the reporter, for his reasons, decided to call me a sports psychologist. But even though my Ph.D. is in sport psychology, I can't call myself a sports psychologist. It's just the rules of the game."

He deals in science, not psychology. Likewise, regular psychologists can't call themselves sports psychologists—and sports psychologists can't call themselves sports scientists.

"You need to differentiate," Beauchamp says. "The public knows nothing about that."

So here you go, public. Now you know.

On to Mindroom.

It's not *Clockwork Orange*. It's sports science. Specifically, a collection of sports-science technology engineered to help athletes get their minds right by working on their bodies. Mental conditioning via physical conditioning. A combination of any number of tools, such as the ones Beauchamp has shown me, Mindroom looks a little different for every client, depending on their needs.

Beauchamp is far from the only sports scientist in the world working with athletes. European soccer clubs are all about it, and have been for the better part of the last decade. Take, for instance, Manchester United, which has a half-dozen or more sports scientists, and Chelsea F.C., which, I've been told, has more than a dozen sports scientists on staff.

"And when we're talking sports scientists in North America," Beauchamp says, "teams may have one sport scientist, and most teams still have zero."

"That must seem insane to guys like you," I say.

"It *is* insane."

North American teams have some catching up to do, especially in the United States, although they *are* starting to. The Golden State Warriors recently hired sports scientists, as have the Seattle Seahawks, the San Antonio Spurs, the Pittsburgh Pirates, and probably more teams that I couldn't identify. But such scientists are still a new concept, like strength and conditioning coaches used to be.

And of course, every sports scientist, and sports-science staff and company, has their own unique methods, but looking at what Beauchamp is doing with Mindroom provides a good idea of what they all try to do.

Some of it is standard psychology and training, exposing athletes to elements that stress them out, such as high-altitude chambers and various other fitness equipment, so they will be calmer in competition. Beauchamp says this encompasses "everything from biomechanics, physiology, to those chambers to swimming pools to underwater cameras to—you name it. RFID technology for monitoring all the athletes on the field. Emotional measurement. Everything."

Beauchamp works with more than fifty companies to produce the equipment he needs. If those companies don't have equipment for something specific Beauchamp wants to do, he'll work with them to design and custom-build it. He's done this several times with one of his primary partners, Thought Technology, one of the world's leading producers of what's known as "biofeedback tech"—basically, equipment that reads various activity in your body, including everything from heart rate to, yes, EEG brain-wave patterns.

Beauchamp's work with Thought Technology is, in large part, where Mindroom began.

On my second day in Montreal, Beauchamp takes me to the Thought Tech office to meet his team of partners; there they teach me not only how much the mind and body truly drive one another but also how, because of that, we as a human race can—and maybe even need—to evolve.

Chapter 8

Rule the Body, Rule the Mind

Thought Tech's office is in a sprawling, plain, gray, warehouse-looking building in LaSalle, a rougher part of the Montreal area. I spend a few hours with Thought Tech founder and president Hal Myers and cofounder and vice president Lawrence Klein—two clean-shaven, gray-haired men inching past middle age, Myers a lean mountain biker, Klein a stocky gym rat—as well as product engineer Marc Saab, a younger guy, balding, bearded, who plays hockey.

They tell me that Mindroom began with a call to the Thought Tech office in 2005. When Klein went to Saab's office to tell him who was on the phone, Saab didn't believe him. It was Bruno Demichelis, a successful sports psychologist for soccer team A.C. Milan.

When the secretary passed along the message, Saab says he thought, *There must be some kind of A.C. Milan in South Shore. Like the Staten Island Yankees, or something.* He said, "A.C. Milan? From Italy? No. Someone mixed up some e-mails. There's no A.C. Milan coming here."

Klein told him, "No, Bruno Demichelis, from A.C. Milan, is coming here."

Saab googled him. *This guy is really coming here?* He still didn't believe it. And then, he says, "He showed up, with bright red pants and a sweater, and he was like, *Brrrrraaaaahhhhh!* And we were like, *Okay, this must be for real.*"

What led Demichelis to Montreal that fateful day? In May 2005, A.C. Milan played Liverpool in the UEFA Champions League championship match in Istanbul. Milan was the heavy favorite and took an instant lead with a goal in the first minute. They took more control throughout the first half, which ended with Milan leading 3–0.

But then a slew of mistakes undid them: Liverpool tied the match in the second half, 3–3, and Milan couldn't close it, their strikers sending one shot on goal after another sailing over the crossbar. The match ended regulation tied 3–3, remained deadlocked throughout extra time, and went to penalties to decide the victor.

Milan's mental mistakes compounded, and unbelievably, Liverpool won penalties, 3–2, and thus, the championship.

Demichelis couldn't take it. So he called.

Klein, Saab, and Demichelis came up with a lab design for Demichelis to take back to Italy, gave him a quote, and off he went. He invited them to visit a year later when the lab was finished, and they loved it. It covered everything from nutrition and physical analysis, but of course, one of its central themes was the mind. Computers with all the equipment and software necessary to analyze an athlete's mind, from heart monitors and galvanic skin-response sensors to, yes, EEG. Demichelis even installed couches covered in Ferrari leather, maybe their favorite detail.

In 2007, A.C. Milan once again found themselves in the UEFA Champions League finals—and once again, they faced none other than Liverpool.

A.C. Milan took the lead, 1–0, in the forty-fifth minute, held on to it going into the half, scored again in the second half, and allowed just one Liverpool goal along the way. No mental lapses, final score 2–1, champions.

"And then," Saab says, "the phones started ringing. The perfect Hollywood ending. And it's boomed since then."

The Vancouver Canucks, who had gone seventeen years without making the Stanley Cup Finals, implemented Mindroom in 2010, made the playoffs as a number one seed, defeated the defending champs, and made the finals, which they took to seven games before losing to the Boston Bruins. Perhaps the most famous and sexy Mindroom buyer: the Ferrari Formula 1 team, which set some records after they started using it. Scores of Olympians began acquiring Mindroom, as well as various divisions of the militaries in both the United States and Canada. There are dozens of teams and athletes, in other words, who use the program—but Beauchamp and the Thought Tech crew swore me to secrecy.

In addition, dozens of elite athletes and organizations such as Tom Brady and the New England Patriots, and the Golden State Warriors, have used, if not the entire Mindroom setup, some of their products and methods.

They all learn to see things in their bodies that were once invisible. As a result, instead of being controlled by their brain, they can take control of their brain, making it work for them and not against them.

So, let's take a closer look at some of what Thought Tech and Mindroom focus on in their work with athletes, which will also show us a lot about humans in general. In short, in a couple of huge ways, our brains have pieces of hardware in them that are out-of-date—meaning that Beauchamp and the Mindroom crew are helping athletes to evolve.

Thought Tech's biggest claim to fame may be Myers's invention of the GSR2, the world's first handheld, portable biofeedback device that can be used by everyone from clinician to stressed-out mom to elite athlete. Autographed pictures with notes of gratitude from celebrities using the device adorn the Thought Technology walls, everyone from Bill Clinton to the pope.

It looks like a computer mouse. You hold it in your left hand and place your index and middle fingers on metal sensors, which then register the galvanic skin response that Beauchamp showed me. The GSR2 tells you how stressed you are simply by playing a dull tone that starts the minute your fingers touch the sensors. The tone rises and falls depending on your stress level.

They demonstrate thusly: Saab hands me a GSR2, tells me how to put it on, then looks me in the eye, intense, and says, "Okay, now I'm going to ask you a very embarrassing question. Get ready."

"Okay, sure," I say, a million possibilities already racing through my head: *Did you really suck so bad in college? Jeez, WHY? And why are you still thinking about it all these years later? Does your wife know you're actually crazy? And she—*

They're all just grinning at me.

"We don't even have to ask the question," Saab says. "You're preparing for the question. Listen to that! You're reacting big-time."

Only then do I realize that the GSR2 tone is noticeably high-pitched and loud.

"That's quicker than any EEG," Beauchamp says with a grin.

"Quicker than anything," Saab says. "Right now your body is deciding whether you should kill all of us."

He explains that we have two nervous systems, the *sensory system*—you know someone's touching your arm because neurons send that message to the brain, and you move your arm because motor neurons tell your arm muscles to contract and move—and then there's the *autonomic* nervous system (ANS), which generally operates automatically, telling your food to digest, your heart to beat, your skin to cool off or heat up, your lungs to breathe. It is in this autonomic nervous system that the sympathetic and parasympathetic systems exist: achieving *homeostasis* means having these two systems balanced with each other. Sympathetic is the gas, parasympathetic the brake.

That GSR2 measured my ANS response, which I was totally unaware of.

Turns out there is a *lot* happening in there—of course—but what athletes need to know is that when that stress kicks in, one of the first things that happens is the adrenal glands on the kidneys start firing up and pumping out adrenaline, activating fight-or-flight mode. "You know what that is," Saab says. "Your ears get hot. You feel your heart beating in your neck. Those are physical manifestations of anxiety and stress. Your brain senses a danger—a saber-toothed tiger, the end of the world, because we evolved from having to fight for our lives."

And at the same time the brake for all of that has been disabled. "That's the key," Saab says, "because that happens in milliseconds." When he put the GSR2 on my hand and said he was going to ask me an embarrassing question, my ANS flooded the engine with gas and cut the brake line. "Everything shoots through the roof and you're raging with adrenaline," Saab says. He says this is called "sympathetic arousal" or "parasympathetic imbalance."

Too much throttle, no brake. "You're jacked," Saab says.

Once this imbalance sets in, you start to sweat more, your blood vessels constrict, which makes your hands cold—hence the term *cold sweat*—and the body concentrates blood flow around the main organs. "So if a bear eats your arm off, you won't die," Saab says. "That's why blood flow is restricted to the core."

Then you get tense. "Think of your golf swing," Saab says. "If you're nervous, your muscles will not behave the same way, and a golf swing has to be fluid."

We've all seen how devastating nerves and tension can be for an athlete. Think of Michigan's Chris Webber calling time-out in the final seconds of the 1993 NCAA Championship game when the team had no time-outs to call, resulting in a technical foul and ultimately a loss. Or the Dallas Cowboys' Tony Romo, fumbling the field goal snap in the 2007 NFC Wild Card playoff game. Or Bill Buckner, the Boston Red Sox first baseman, letting the ground ball go through his legs in the 1986 World Series game six. And so on.

Some of Thought Tech and Mindroom's primary clients are Olympic athletes, and Olympians perform under perhaps the most enormous pressure in all of sports. Four years of training and meticulous self-sacrificing in preparation for an event that can last as few as thirty seconds—and in front of millions of people, maybe billions. "The pinnacle of pressure," Saab says. "And it applies to anybody performing under pressure. So having to give a speech you're not prepared for in front of two thousand people is a similar kind of pressure."

A hyperstrong stress response was useful for us humans back in the days of saber-toothed tigers and the constant looming end of the world and need to fight for our lives. And now it's still helpful, especially for athletes—it wakes the mind up and gets its engine roaring. But it can also easily hijack you. "Now, what we do," Saab says, "unfortunately, is we're ten minutes late for a meeting and we're having a similar response—which is far too much activity for walking into a meeting. You don't need to scale the wall or kill somebody with your bare hands. You don't need all of that going on, but that's what your body is doing. And that's just naturally unevolved, right? You don't *need* that response. So your body's preparing you for something that is not going to happen."

I hadn't even thought of this until he said the words *naturally unevolved*. How often have I freaked out and either been paralyzed with fear or—my worst response—burst into an angry temper? I realize, in this moment, that all I am doing there is allowing my base instincts to take over, which might be perfectly fine if I were in *The Walking Dead* facing down a zombie horde, but isn't exactly useful for disagreements or for meeting deadlines.

Saab doesn't say this because it's too grandiose, but one thing Mindroom is doing, then, is pushing athletes forward in human evolution. "The mental, emotional, and physical are inseparable," he says. "You have a thought, you have an emotion, it has a physiological manifestation."

Saab thinks that athletes often have no idea just how much their thoughts and emotions affect their body. "Thoughts and emotions actually change how your body acts," he says. "If you don't realize you're physiologically reacting, that your body is reacting differently, you're doing things your body normally doesn't do. You can be stiff, you can limit your range of motion. Imagine a golfer—how come he can hit a hundred putts in a row when he's practicing, but when it's down to the eighteenth green on Sunday, he misses and it lips out? We know his shoulders are not acting the way they normally act. He's tensing up. But he thinks, *Oh well, it was mental.*"

The "mental" creates something physical, and controlling the physical can take control of the mental. When athletes work with the likes of Beauchamp and Thought Tech, they create the linkage between the mental and the physical.

This is so important because, as Saab puts it, "Once you start making mistakes, that leads to all the negative self-talk and anxiety and doubt, and all of a sudden you're in a loop where, when you re-create those thoughts and encourage those thoughts, you've strengthened that emotional physiological impairment."

In other words, you choke.

Beauchamp dislikes that term—*choke, choking,* etc.—and even the term *impairment*. He's found in his research and work over the years that spinning in a positive direction works better for athletes, so he says stuff like "just getting in your own way."

To walk through the basics of how Beauchamp and his colleagues do this, they tell me about a guy I'll call Jack. He was a young up-and-comer who'd just signed his first NHL contract. The Mindroom crew had been working with him for about five days, with Beauchamp teaching him breathing techniques and running other tests on him. They show me twelve minutes of data they recorded from their work with Jack one day—galvanic skin response, skin conductance, sweat response, breathing rates, skin temperature, heart rate, and tension in his shoulders and trapezius muscles.

First, they did some warm-ups with him. Crossword puzzles, stuff like that. Jack's breathing was steady and clean, the data showing smooth cresting and falling lines, like waves rolling into the beach. Jack's skin temperature and muscle tension, too, were smooth as can be. "Rhythmic," Saab says, "with a certain cleanliness to them."

Then they had Jack do serial sevens—"some bullshit math," Saab calls it.

To demonstrate, he makes me do it, too: "Start at one thousand and eighty-one and subtract seven, out loud, and do them as fast as you can, and I'll correct you when you make a mistake."

Two subtractions later, I'm already struggling.

"How much fun are you having?" Saab asks.

"None whatsoever."

He laughs. "Right! It's not fun at all. And what you don't know is that your body is reacting to that, because we're all sitting here; we know the test. You're like, *Why is this guy making me do math right now? Do I look stupid?* And all of a sudden you get that feeling."

Saab had mercy on me. We only did serial sevens for maybe ten seconds. Poor Jack, though—Saab made him go for three minutes. And, Saab says, "Look what happens." The instant they began, Jack's data went haywire. His breathing fell apart, his heart rate went jagged, his skin temperature plummeted, and most striking of all, his shoulders became almost painfully tense.

And Jack noticed *none* of this, nor showed any obvious physical signs.

After that, they switched Jack to a computer task, using a mouse to move a circle into a square. That's it. But Saab kept messing with him, intentionally making it harder than it needed to be and telling Jack he was doing worse than he really was. "Athletes want to know right away, 'What'd the other guys get?'" Saab says. "'What's a good score?'" He told Jack something like five hundred, when really, it's impossible to score one hundred. And Jack scored thirty.

Just sitting there, not physically doing anything, he tensed his shoulders for six straight minutes.

"So at this point," Saab says, "he's like, *Screw this guy, man. Screw this whole thing.* But he's already hooked up, and like you've said, that's a weird feeling. He's already in the chair. He's not going anywhere. And look at what he does."

Jack almost completely stopped breathing.

When he did breathe, he wasn't taking the deep, resonant breaths he needed, but instead, short and quick. "He goes into a slight panic," Saab says. "Just trying to move a freaking mouse."

Jack's muscles remained supertense, too.

When this happens—short, quick breaths, tense muscles—the rest of the body activates its stress response automatically. The adrenal glands activate, fight-or-flight activates, panic sets in. "And," Saab adds, "that takes energy, by the way. So you're fatiguing yourself for no good reason. Total waste. If you're the golfer, you're not moving your arms the way you're supposed to move your arms."

Beauchamp says that different people exhibit different symptoms. "Some athletes show a lot of muscle tension. Others will show a lot of skin conductance. Others will hold their breath. So you need to find, individually, what are the symptoms of stress on an individual level? And this allows us to do that. Because in short, when athletes get tense, they slow down."

They run like they're hauling a piano, their bat speed slows down, their golf drives veer left or right, their hockey sticks feel they're swinging anvils. "Cement hands," Saab calls it. And hockey players, when this happens, Saab says, they'll say things like, "Oh, I'm just holding the stick too tight." He adds, "You have a way of rationalizing what it is—but we can identify *exactly* what it is."

Baseball players trying to make a throw, Beauchamp says while grinning at me, can get the Yips.

He's right—remember how my shoulder, and eventually my whole body, felt stuck? Muscle tension.

All of that is the body's extreme stress response kicking into high gear—and all the while the athlete has no idea it's happening.

That's the bad news. The good news is that it is something athletes can learn to manage.

That takes some work, though: when Saab finally let him stop, by then, Jack was angry. Saab showed him the data and asked, "How do you think this affects your performance?"

Jack shrugged. "What is that?"

"Oh, that's your muscle tension."

"But I wasn't tense."

"This shows that you were. You were contracting your traps for six minutes."

"No, I wasn't," Jack said, angrier still. "I maybe flinched. But I didn't *hold* them for six minutes."

Beauchamp and Saab put Jack through more training. Beauchamp told Jack to flex his traps as hard as he could for several seconds, then drop his shoulders and exhale. As Jack exhaled, Beauchamp put his hands on Jack's shoulders and pushed down, telling him, "Exhale, exhale, exhale. Drop and drop and drop."

They kept doing this until the levels on the screen showed Jack's heart rate, breathing frequency, and muscle tension bottom out.

Then they asked how he felt.

"Okay," Jack said. "That feels great."

"Better, right?" Saab said.

Then Jack got real. "Yeah, but when am I gonna do that?"

Recounting the story, Saab is blunt, saying, "He had that voice. Like, *Okay, Coach told me to do this, so I'm doing it, but when am I gonna do this for real?* And you can imagine an athlete thinking like that, probably not with us, but after he leaves. His buddy asks, 'What did you think?' 'Ah, it was bullshit. Let's get a hamburger.'"

Saab told Jack, "Well, you're not gonna walk around like that, but let me ask you something. If you have one second to make a decision—if you have to stop the puck from getting out of the zone, and take a slap shot, and you have one second to do it, would you rather be loose, or would you rather be tight?"

"Loose. I'd rather be loose."

"Well, how do you think you're doing over here?"

Jack didn't know what to say.

"That's when, all of a sudden, the athlete can't talk his way out of it," Saab says. "It makes perfect sense."

From there, men and women like Jack learn how to analyze every part of their performance in new ways. On the bench, are they building their energy back up and keeping focus—or are they stressing out? Are they breathing well, or are they huffing and puffing? In the last ten minutes, have they been feeling good—or are they exhausted?

Beauchamp says that every athlete, whether they realize it or not, has two ways of warming up: "general dynamic" and "specific." Beauchamp uses methods like those I just described with Jack to teach athletes how to use their breathing before—and during—the games to make sure they are ready. Beauchamp and his colleagues use the psychophysiology to teach it, and then they show them how to integrate that knowledge into their routines. Seamless. "If they're doing this as a warm-up routine," Beauchamp says, "then you can guarantee that when they start their competition, they're much more ready to go."

Sports scientists like the Mindroom crew show athletes how their body creates stress they don't even know is there, and then how to do something about it. Saab says, "To be able to have a thought and have the signal change on the screen, that's a jump, right? You can connect someone up, and in five minutes show them how to change their heart rate." And, he's saying, that means changing their mental state. "That's science fiction, right? But we do it all the time."

Something else the Mindroom crew does, entirely by means of breathing, is they not only help athletes get ready to go, but also help them calm down enough after games so that they can actually get some good sleep.

No performance-enhancing drug or piece of technology can

compare to a good night's sleep. When we sleep, a flood of cerebrospinal fluid flows through the brain and clears out waste proteins and toxins that build up between neurons while we're awake. Dr. Maiken Nedergaard, the codirector of the University of Rochester Department of Neurosurgery and a professor of neurology and neuroscience who published a sleep study in *Science,* told NPR, "It's like a dishwasher."

Except much more complex: not only does the fluid flush toxins, but your neurons also shrink a bit, allowing the fluid to move freely through the brain. When you wake up, neurons expand again, and the cerebrospinal fluid eases on out. "Almost like opening and closing a faucet," Nedergaard told NPR. "It's that dramatic."

While it would be nice if our brains could clear those toxic proteins while we're awake, too, Nedergaard told NPR he thinks they don't because this cleaning uses a lot of energy, and says he doesn't think the brain is capable of both cleaning itself while also handling all the sensory input we receive while awake.

Athletes might not know all the science behind it, but this is likely why they are getting really into taking naps before games. A little sleep is hugely refreshing.

A few years ago, the *New York Times* ran a feature about the pregame naps of star basketball players, hockey players, and baseball players. Then NBA deputy commissioner Adam Silver—now the league commissioner—told the paper, "Everyone in the league office knows not to call players at 3 P.M."

Of course, somehow, there's a stigma around this as well. *Boston Globe* columnist Alex Beam in January 2016 published a ranty piece about all the napping, saying that it was just "beauty rest" and, in his words, another sign of "the prissification of the modern athlete." This is inaccurate on its face, but it's also hilariously blind: Boston's own teams have been winning in part *because* of said beauty rest, which has been thoroughly documented. Before the Boston Bruins played game seven of the 2011 Stanley Cup Finals, Brigham and Women's Hospital sleep expert Dr. Charles Czeisler told the team to skip their morning practice and sleep in. The Bruins won the game 4–0 to claim the Cup. Then, in 2013, Czeisler persuaded the Boston Red Sox to turn a Fenway Park room into a nap room; the Sox won the World Series that season.

Beauty rest? More like . . . *beastly* rest.

(Sorry.)

As you might expect, however, convincing these athletes to try woo-woo-sounding breathing techniques to get better sleep isn't always easy. For example, Brandon Parsons, the clinical deputy director at Neurodezign (yes, that's how they spell it) was part of a Mindroom team that went to Vancouver in 2010 to work with the Canucks.

They set up shop in a little room off to the side of the Canucks' home locker room, and they had about five minutes to explain what they were doing to the team. That wasn't enough to really sell them on it. "As a high-level athlete, you know yourself, and these guys are solicited all the time," Parsons says. "Everybody wants their time, everybody wants their attention, and they just see everything as a distraction, or an annoyance, or something more they have to do during their day, and their hours, especially during the season, are full. So the big challenge is to get these guys in the room to begin with."

Parsons decided to target a couple of their leaders. He can't tell me individual names—and the Canucks didn't respond to my requests for interviews—but Parsons could tell me about his experience with one of the team leaders, and how it changed everything. We'll call the guy Chief. "One of the guys who was kind of against what we were doing . . ." Parsons says. "He had more of a negative personality, he was still a leader in the room who the guys tended to follow. So I specifically went after him."

Parsons went to Chief one day and said, "Okay, take me through what a game day looks like for you."

Chief talked him through his usual routines and how he felt and all, and it was nothing out of the ordinary, but then he said what Parsons hears all the time from top athletes: "I don't feel rested the next day. I don't feel like I sleep well."

Parsons says, "Athletes in general absolutely suck at being able to shut off after a game. They go home, it's eleven thirty, midnight, and their brain's still wired, still going a hundred miles per hour. And they gotta calm down and relax."

Usually they play video games or watch TV until they get tired, though the problem with that is that such activities only keep the brain awake, and they pass out because they burn out, not because they're settling into restful sleep. This makes their sleep far less useful than it should be because their brain and their body don't fully recover, and they wake up tired.

Worse, some use a couple of drinks to conk out, and alcohol generally ruins sleep.

Chief told Parsons that he avoids drinking but he usually ends up playing Xbox for an hour or two before he can fall asleep. Parsons explained why this doesn't do him much good, and then said, "After the next game, come see me. We'll do five minutes of mindful breathing, and that's it. I guarantee you'll sleep the best night you've had all season."

Chief agreed, but then after the next game, he tried talking his way out of it. "Man, I'm *tired*," he said. "I just want to go home, I've got my wife and kids—I just want to go home."

"Five minutes," Parsons said. "You can afford five minutes. If it doesn't work, you never have to come again, and I won't bug you."

Chief said okay. Parsons hooked him up to a computer, same as Beauchamp had me, and used the same program that Beauchamp used, with the sensors and the breathing pacer, and helped Chief find his ideal breathing rate. That ended up being six breaths per minute, four seconds inhaling, six seconds exhaling. After five minutes of that, Parsons unhooked him and asked how he felt.

"That's it?" Chief said. "You really think that's gonna help me sleep? You're nuts."

"Come back and see me tomorrow morning," Parsons said. "And let me know."

Chief went home, and Parsons went to his hotel, where it was his turn to not sleep. He tossed and turned all night, nervous as he'd ever been, hoping Chief was sleeping well. If he was, then he was in, and others would follow—but if Chief wasn't sleeping well, Parsons was screwed. "We may as well close all our doors," he says. "Because, again, these guys are very reticent. And the guys who are young, they're a little easier to get in, because they're new and they're green and they're looking for anything to get the edge, but they're still going to follow their leaders, so I was really hoping to get this guy."

After his sleepless night, Parsons returned to the office the next morning.

Chief was already there, waiting for him. "I don't know what the hell you did to me," he said, "but you were right. I slept better than I've slept every single night. What's that system? I want to buy one so I can take it on the road with me."

After that, Parsons had guys lined up to see him.

Chapter 9

This Is Your Brain on Drugs

The world of sports is littered with stories of men and women partaking of substances—some legal, some less legal—to catapult themselves into one desired mind-set or another. That's why big-league ballplayers will play with a wad of dip in their lips, and why, after winning the Super Bowl in 2016, Peyton Manning said he was going to "drink a lot of Budweiser," and why it seems all of us are addicted to our morning coffee.

Long before sports science became a thing, athletes had been using all manner of drugs for everything from getting up for the game, to coping with injury, to just getting sleep. In this chapter, I wade through what modern science has to show about some of them.

Of course, this rabbit hole is enormous, a chapter that could easily become its own book. For our purposes, I'm not getting into prescription pharmaceuticals such as Ritalin and Adderall, beta-blockers, amphetamines, and the like; nor will I get into anything that's outright illegal, like cocaine or heroin. Basically, I've left out anything banned by WADA (the World Anti-Doping Agency), the USADA (the U.S. Anti-Doping Agency), and other governing bodies of sport. I'm making one exception, for marijuana, for reasons that will soon become clear. As for the rest, I'm focusing on the most popular drugs—alcohol, nicotine, caffeine, and marijuana—as well as one nootropic product, a "smart drug" that is actually not banned, and has been scientifically tested.

And look, be smart and talk with your doctors before diving into any sort of drug use, okay?

CAFFEINE

This is the world's most popular psychoactive performance-enhancing drug by far: according to some estimates, about 90 percent of adults in the United States drink coffee every day. And in fact, caffeine was on the World Anti-Doping Agency's banned list until 2004. Of course, of all the things athletes endorse, as far as I could find, coffee is rarely one of them—although there is Matthew Dellavedova, the NBA point guard from Australia who plays like a Jack Russell terrier. After the 2015 NBA Finals, when it was revealed that Delly—then playing with the Cleveland Cavaliers—pounded coffee before and even during games, he got his own brew, called G'Day Mate, from the Cleveland Coffee Company.

Beyond coffee, elite athletes get their caffeine fix a number of ways. In 2011, Major League Baseball even grew concerned about the sharp rise in energy drink consumption after the league banned amphetamines in 2005. One pitcher, Wesley Wright of the Houston Astros, ended up hospitalized with dehydration in 2009 after drinking several cans of Red Bull and other sodas before a game.

Of course, lots of athletes are sponsored by and drink Red

Bull and other energy drinks and do quite well. The hundreds of Red Bull–sponsored athletes include everyone from Olympic and X Games champions to Anthony Davis, the New Orleans Pelicans power forward who was the 2012 NCAA Player of the Year. Monster, the world's second-most-popular energy drink, has been endorsed by plenty of big-name athletes, including UFC champs Conor McGregor and Ronda Rousey, as well as New England Patriots tight end Rob Gronkowski.

And for good reason. Caffeine is a *stimulant,* and its effect comes largely from how it interacts with the neurotransmitter *adenosine.* Adenosine binds with neurons to slow them down, which makes you sleepy, and it dilates blood vessels, which helps the body stay good and oxygenated during sleep. Caffeine is an *adenosine-receptor antagonist,* binding to adenosine receptors and thus leaving fewer receptors for *actual* adenosine to bind to, meaning you don't get as sleepy.

Caffeine also activates neural circuits that cause the pituitary gland to give off hormones, which then leads to the creation of adrenaline. This makes you more focused and gives you more energy, which is basically why we all drink coffee—but it can also seriously backfire for those of us prone to anxiety. Plus, like almost any other drug, caffeine can create a physical dependency—within a day or two of not having coffee, about half of people will feel headaches, nausea, and sleepiness. Also, caffeine, like most drugs, increases dopamine production in the brain, and dopamine is one of the primary reasons why any of us get addicted to anything.

NICOTINE

I've dipped exactly two times in my life. I regret both. Once was during a baseball practice in college, which didn't do anything for me that day except make me more anxious. (Back then, my obsession with honoring God—or maybe just my narcissism— compelled me to connect my every action to the eternal fate of the universe via my soul.) The second time, I took it while playing the video game *Call of Duty*. I'm okay at first-person shooter games, but not great, and that night I was extra bad. I was getting ten kills a game at best, dying twice as often. Not the ideal gamer teammate.

One of my buddies was dipping and swore by the stuff, and he was basically getting the inverse of my stats if not way better, so I said screw it, let me try.

Ten minutes later, rampage. Even better stats than my buddy.

Ten minutes after that, I was bent over the rails of our dorm balcony about to puke.

Aside from a few regrettable nights when a couple drinks too many compelled me to have a cigarette, and a few cigars with buddies here or there, I pretty much avoided all things nicotine since then. Now I regret that, too, because like most people, when I thought "nicotine" I thought cigarettes and tobacco. Those are just delivery systems, though. Nicotine itself is, in many ways, quite the beautiful drug.

Nicotine binds to an acetylcholine receptor—the *nicotinic receptor*—and creates an artificial supply of acetylcholine. In small doses, it can be wonderful, both calming you down and getting you focused and motivated. Nicotine users can develop a tolerance, however, and in larger doses, it will create an artificial acetylcholine deficiency. (This is why, for instance, cigarette addicts need a cigarette so badly after waking up in the morning, why they need a fresh fix every few hours, and why the cigarette addict without a cigarette is such a nightmare to be around.)

Nicotine is also highly addictive for the same reason most other drugs are: it activates our reward pathways, giving our brains nice big shots of dopamine.

Cigarettes, of course, are the most common way to get a nicotine fix, though athletes typically get theirs via chewing tobacco and dip. Smoking cigarettes on the field of play basically never happens (except in *The Replacements,* the football movie starring Keanu Reeves that features the character Nigel Gruff, a British kicker who takes the field puffing away). Dip and chewing tobacco—sometimes lumped together as "spit tobacco"—are, of course, staples in baseball, despite long-term efforts by Major League Baseball to curb their use. Spit tobacco was so common in the nineties that, in 1998, MLB allowed the nonprofit National Spit Tobacco Education Program (NSTEP) to perform oral exams on 141 players during spring training. More than 80 of those players—about 59 percent—had lesions or soft-tissue damage in their mouths because of spit tobacco use, 15 of them so seriously that the players had to get biopsied.

Chipper Jones, the now-retired Atlanta Braves legendary third baseman, is just one example of the baseball player who's been unable to kick his dip habit. He started dipping when he was fourteen, and as long ago as 1997, he was talking about wanting to quit. In 2001, during one of many attempts to quit, Jones went into a gnarly slump, 7-for-45. "I fly off the handle at the least little thing," he said. "I feel like I'm always tensed up, never relaxed, edgy . . . It's scary when you try to lick it and find out it's this difficult. It has a very large grip."

And as recently as April 2016, well into retirement, Jones appeared on camera for an interview at a charity golf tournament, and he still had a big wad in his lip.

Thing is, cigarettes and dip are only delivery methods for nicotine—the only major risk of nicotine itself is addiction. The problem for these baseball guys—and anyone else addicted to tobacco—is the cancer-causing nature of tobacco. They could still get their nicotine fix other ways.

And nicotine is ideal for the athlete. Soon as the brain gets a nicotine hit, you feel a nice kick as the drug activates your adrenal glands, resulting in a discharge of epinephrine—that is, adrenaline. That kick ripples through the rest of the body by sparking a sudden release of glucose, a primary source of fuel for the brain, and by increasing blood pressure, heart rate, and respiration. How strong this hits depends on how anxious you are and the strength of the nicotine dose. In general, cigarettes contain roughly ten milligrams, about two of which make it into your bloodstream— but the numbers on chewing tobacco and dip are pretty much impossible to estimate.

The safest ways to get nicotine are gum and nicotine patches. I wish I'd considered them back in my college days. A few years ago, I worked with a guy who went through a pack of nicotine gum a day, trying to kick his own old dip habit—he was a former ballplayer, too. He offered me some of the gum when I told him I'd never tried it, and I liked it. It got me focused and alert and calm all at once. I still use it during harder workdays, when I need a little extra help focusing. I've also even tried it out during softball and pickup basketball a couple times. I don't use it very often because I don't want to be dependent upon it, but if I'd known how convenient, useful, and relatively harmless nicotine gum was back in my college days, I think I would have used it quite a bit.

ALCOHOL

A few beers might make someone better at golf, but beyond that, alcohol as performance enhancer has long since been debunked, for obvious reasons. A few Budweisers after winning a Super Bowl are beautiful, and sure, a drink or two can increase alpha-brain-wave activity, which will make you more relaxed, and which *typically* makes you feel better. But there are too many negative side effects.

For starters, even a few drinks at night can have lingering detrimental effects the following day. Urban Meyer famously chased sleeping pills with beer every night during his time of great stress a few years ago, and he still only got four hours of sleep a night. Grabbing a drink will chill you out, sure, but it can wreck your sleep.

Alcohol *will* help you fall asleep faster, but it's going to be garbage sleep compared to being sober. Alcohol weakens the REM phase of sleep, which happens about ninety minutes after we drift off, and, as the phase that does the most work to restore us, is the most important part of sleep. More than two dozen studies indicate that disrupting REM sleep leads to drowsiness and concentration problems the next day. Remember, from chapter eight, how sleep acts as a sort of "dishwasher" for the brain, clearing it of toxins and waste? When we can't get enough good, restful sleep for this to happen, that old waste gets in the way.

Particularly important, in regard to sleep and alcohol in general, is a neurotransmitter known as GABA (or *gamma-aminobutyric acid*). We have "excitatory" and "inhibitory" neurotransmitters that drive communication in the brain. I think of them as "go" and "stop" signals. Go signals tell neurons to fire off more go signals. Stop signals shut them down.

And GABA is the most important stop drug in our central nervous system. When neurons receive GABA, they're told to stop sending new signals until a go drug comes along. Alcohol increases GABA activity in the brain, which is why it's so relaxing at first. Neurons more prone to sending and receiving GABA can be found in parts of the brain responsible for generating what's called "slow-wave sleep," the most important stage of REM sleep. (These make up the *brain-stem reticular activating system,* a relatively unconscious part of the brain that manages wakefulness and transitioning between being awake and asleep; the *thalamus,* which plays a role in our ability to voluntarily move our body; the *hypothalamus,* which produces hormones that govern circadian rhythm, sleep, and body temperature, plus thirst, hunger, mood, and sex drive; and the *basal forebrain,* a group of parts working with Big Fronty to produce acetylcholine, which also makes the brain more awake and alert.)

Then there's how alcohol affects another neurotransmitter, *glutamate,* which, as our brain's most important go drug, is essentially the opposite of GABA. Glutamate wakes neurons up; GABA shuts them down. And basically, as a *glutamate antagonist,* alcohol gets in glutamate's way.

All of this contributes to how alcohol tends to make people sluggish, slurred, and sleepy.

This kind of relaxation—and copious amounts of GABA—can actually be wonderful for your body, but excess alcohol has a way of running wild with it all and hijacking the brain's natural systems in an unhealthy way.

And beyond the problems it causes with sleep, alcohol is dangerous on a larger level: it is one of the most addictive substances on earth, and it can change the brain not unlike hard, illegal drugs such as cocaine and heroin.

Essentially, alcohol hijacks the brain in order to make the brain want more of it.

Some brains are more vulnerable to this than others. About a decade ago, Dr. David Belin and Dr. Barry Everitt, professors in the department of pharmacology at the University of Cambridge, showed that some people are far more prone to addiction than the average person: some people more easily become hooked on a drug like cocaine, and then they literally cannot stop themselves from seeking out more of it. They cannot control their brain, and it's not their fault. Testing this theory on rats, the doctors found that 20 percent of the rats kept going back for more cocaine even when they started receiving painful electric shocks.

They also found that alcohol addiction in particular is connected to what they call "waiting impulsivity." In other words, the more a person drinks, the less patience he has—even when sober. This means that a sober person who drinks frequently may still be highly vulnerable to making ill-advised, compulsive choices driven by irrational impulse. As an athlete, this would be especially problematic.

That said, Belin and Everitt also found that this compulsiveness subsides when one stops drinking.

CANNABIS

Here's where I break my rule of not discussing anything illegal (or, in this case, illegal-ish), because—well, for just one of many examples, look at the story of Jim McMahon.

It's been a long twenty years since McMahon retired in 1996, and even longer since he won the 1986 Super Bowl with the Chicago Bears. At fifty-seven, he has long suffered from chronic pain wrought by countless injuries over his fifteen-year career, including a broken neck and more concussions than he can remember. McMahon has also already been diagnosed with dementia, and he gets awful headaches, battles clinical depression, and struggles with his memory, vision, and ability to speak. To cope, McMahon was prescribed Percocet, the narcotic, opioid painkiller. It numbed his pain, but it also left him in a mental fog, and like many who use opioid painkillers, he got addicted, to the tune of one hundred pills per *month*. "Doing more harm than good," he told the *Chicago Tribune* in January 2016.

Percocet contains oxycodone, the basis for OxyContin, one of the most prescribed painkillers in America. Oxycodone, an opioid, isn't much different from heroin. A single dose of oxy commonly creates debilitating cravings for more, and causes users to experience withdrawal symptoms on par with those of heroin addicts. Two million Americans abused or were dependent on prescription opioids, according to a 2014 CDC report. The CDC also reports that prescription opioids killed more than 165,000 people between 1999 and 2014. This is what killed Prince.

McMahon started using medical marijuana after his home state of Arizona legalized it in 2010. "A godsend," he calls it. He smokes it in the morning to get out of bed, in the afternoon if he's feeling a need, and before bed to help him sleep. And he hasn't needed Percocet in years.

McMahon's is just one of many similar stories. Some reports estimate that more than 50 percent of NFL players smoke regularly.

One assistant football coach recently told Bleacher Report's Mike Freeman, "If you tested players during the season every week, we wouldn't be able to field a league. We'd have to merge with the [Canadian Football League]."

Ricky Williams, a great NFL running back before he failed multiple drug tests in the early 2000s and retired early, has said that cannabis works "ten times better than Paxil" for his social anxiety disorder. That's why he began smoking weed in the first place.

A veteran NFL linebacker told Freeman that smoking weed helped him heal from a concussion faster and with fewer side effects, and it extended his playing career—and helped stave off the suicidal thoughts suffered by teammates and league friends after head injuries.

Mark Stepnoski played thirteen years in the NFL, made five

consecutive Pro Bowls, and won two Super Bowl rings, all after being not just a football All-American in college, but also an academic All-American. After retiring in 2001, he became a spokesman for the National Organization for the Reform of Marijuana Laws. "After a game, you hurt so much, you need something to relax," he once told *Sports Illustrated*. "I'd rather smoke than take painkillers."

Science hasn't studied cannabis's effect on concussion recovery yet, but doctors themselves recommend it, in general, for headaches, sleeplessness, light sensitivity, and loss of appetite—all frequent concussion symptoms—and athletes say weed does more for them than any other painkillers or treatment. Lester Grinspoon, a Harvard emeritus professor of psychiatry, in February 2014 published a letter at *Vice* the headline of which put his argument simply: "The NFL Should Combat Concussions with Cannabis."

This reaches beyond football, too. Former basketball player Jay Williams, who was also saved from a painkiller addiction by cannabis, has said that 80 percent of players in the NBA smoke regularly. Even the U.S. government has filed a patent (number 6630507) for cannabis. They label it "a neuroprotectant" and say that it can limit neurological damage following brain trauma. Marijuana has also been found to effectively block pain signals in the brain and reduce inflammation.

Frank Lucido, a physician in Berkeley who works with NFL players, recently told the *Wall Street Journal* that weed was perfect for treating common sports-related ailments, such as orthopedic pain, brain injury, and depression. He also said, "Marijuana should not be a banned substance. It has too many medical benefits."

One NFL owner told Freeman outright, "Many of us are behind the times."

Indeed, even seeing a football player walk into a weed shop

freaks owners out. Running back Ezekiel Elliott, selected by the Dallas Cowboys as the number four pick in the 2016 draft, caused a stir come preseason when he visited a marijuana dispensary in Seattle, where recreational use is legal. Marijuana use remains forbidden by the NFL, however, and even though Elliott left without buying anything, Cowboys owner Jerry Jones lost it. "It's not good," he told the *Fort Worth Star-Telegram*. "It's just not good."

Early last year, while in Portland for research, I went to one such marijuana dispensary.

The place was nicer than a lot of pharmacies. Classy, sleek, modern, with a warm color palette, mostly white and gray backdrops with splashes of green and orange. There were dozens of different strains displayed in glass cases, as well as shelves of pre-rolled cone joints on the walls.

Between talking with the "budtenders" and looking over research they pointed me to, I was surprised at the complex nature of marijuana. There's a certain beauty to it. The plant is made up of five hundred chemicals that affect the brain via "the entourage effect"—all the chemicals work best together. The two strongest, primary chemicals are tetrahydrocannabinol (THC) and cannabidiol (CBD). THC, the psychoactive component, produces the high, but also does much more: THC has been found to generate exceptional results in relieving pain and arthritis, and in giving chemo patients an appetite.

As for CBD, a 2011 study by physiopathologists and pediatricians in Spain found that when it was given to pigs with brain injuries, CBD sparked their brains' electrical activity back to almost normal levels while also dramatically reducing their stress. In addition, CBD given to mice led to fewer neurons dying in their brains, and CBD has shown potential as an antioxidant.

Of course, like any drug, marijuana has its share of potential side effects. Increased heart rate, increased appetite, dizziness, confusion, paranoia. It's a bad idea for anyone younger than their twenties, in particular, to regularly use cannabis because their brains still have to develop so much more. Studies also show that heavy use—like smoking all day every day—*can* negatively affect IQ, alertness, short-term memory, and reaction time.

That said, research has also found weed to be less dangerous than alcohol and OxyContin—and it's not even close. A six-year study by the United Kingdom Drug Policy Commission concluded that weed was every bit as dangerous as . . . junk food.

Cannabis is not physically addictive, and the risk of developing a tolerance or experiencing withdrawal is relatively minor. Alcohol and opioids, by comparison, are two of the most highly addictive—and destructive—substances on earth. According to the CDC, alcohol poisoning kills six people *per day* on average, and in the United States, excessive alcohol use has led to about eighty-eight thousand deaths and the loss of 2.5 million years of potential life. Meanwhile, among the thirty-three million Americans estimated to have used weed in the past year, there has been a stunning number of resulting deaths: zero.

And as for me, weed helps my anxiety and OCD more than the medication I take, and with far fewer gnarly side effects.

This is going to sound like B.S., but the one time I got high in college, it was an accident. My sophomore year, riding around town shooting video with a classmate for a project, I didn't realize he'd hotboxed his car because I had no idea what hotboxing even was. I caught a secondhand buzz, and then, after he dropped me off at my dorm, I went to practice—and I had one of the best afternoons of my life. Hit great, played great, and best of all, had *zero* worries about throwing. (The next day when that was all gone, I freaked out again, and of course, this is totally unscientific, because I could see a bad high making me paranoid and mentally paralyzed.)

Doctors used to prescribe cannabis to the tune of three *million* prescriptions per year in the 1920s. Until 1943, when physicians were no longer allowed to prescribe cannabis, the U.S. *Pharmacopeia*—the national encyclopedia for medical drugs, basically—listed cannabis as an active ingredient in dozens of medications treating everything from migraines to menstrual cramps. When the government criminalized cannabis, they did so in direct opposition to the American Medical Association, which recommended that it remain legal.

So yeah, since I was already there in a dispensary, and it was legal, I wasn't leaving Portland without trying *something*.

There are two different species of cannabis plant: *Cannabis indica* and *Cannabis sativa.* In short, as the budtenders explained to me, the *indica* strains give you a more mellow "body" buzz great for relaxation, while the *sativas* give you a more heady, "cerebral, uplifting" high, also great for relaxing but also remaining productive. (That is a bit of an overgeneralization—either one, depending on the particular strain of bud you choose, *can* give you the inverse—but that's going to be true more often than not.)

I chose an indica blend called Blue City Diesel. Cost eight bucks. My budtender, a girl with blond dreadlocks wearing a tie-dyed shirt and white tank top, recommended starting with half the joint since I rarely smoke.

I walked around the neighborhood of my Airbnb and carefully smoked exactly half, and stared at the stars.

I chose well. I skipped my medication that night, had a productive night of writing, finished the joint the next morning before flying out, skipped my morning pills, too, and still felt healthy all day. The juxtaposition between how that made me feel versus how, say, drinking made me feel was remarkable. Drinking not only costs more money, but has more than once—particularly during my Years of Madness and Regret—left me waking up feeling just horrible. Not to sound too much like a marijuana fanboy or anything, but by comparison, that little bit left me feeling like my mind had gotten a good massage.

It's hard to believe that in August 2016, the DEA decided to keep marijuana a Schedule I drug, meaning they consider it as dangerous as heroin, despite the fact that heroin kills countless scores of people every year. The only death remotely connected to cannabis use by those aforementioned thirty-three million who partook last year occurred when a guy ate six times the standard serving of a marijuana edible, then decided he needed to jump from a fourth-floor balcony. Tragic, to be sure. But to be clear, the typical headlines after someone ingests too much weed go a little more like this one from an August 2016 *Omaha World-Herald:* "Omaha Dad Finds Pot Brownies, Eats 4 of Them, Says Mean Things to Cat."

NOOTROPICS

Nootropics, aka "smart drugs" and/or supplements that supposedly boost brain function, are rising in popularity among Silicon Valley and CEO types, and nootropics as an overall topic could take an entire book itself. There's research being done on a prominent nootropic called modafinil that makes you smarter, more focused, all that—but it's only available in the U.S. by prescription, and besides, like Adderall and beta blockers, it, too, is banned by the World Anti-Doping Association.

Between the number of banned substances and the murkiness of the science behind most of them, I didn't think I'd look into nootropics when I started exploring all of This Stuff. After all, one of the great sci-fi wishes of all time is to pop a pill and become way better at, well, everything, and unsavory business folk have been making such empty promises for decades. Didn't seem worth getting into.

But then I came across Alpha BRAIN, an all-natural nootropic supplement produced by Onnit, a young supplement and lifestyle company based in Austin, Texas, which several elite athletes openly endorse. There's Houston Texans linebacker Brian Cushing, a team captain, former first-round pick, the NFL's 2009 Defensive Rookie of the Year, a 2009 Pro Bowl selection, and a 2011 All-Pro. In his endorsement at Onnit.com, he says, "Every morning I take Alpha BRAIN. This product keeps me focused in season and out. It has helped me tremendously in my day to day routine."

Chicago Blackhawks star Duncan Keith also appears on the Onnit website saying, "Hockey is not only physically but also mentally demanding. Alpha BRAIN helps my alertness on the ice." Also appearing there are rally driver Ken Block, MMA fighter Tim Kennedy, and Olympic decathlete medalist Trey Hardee. The Onnit company launched in July 2011 with Alpha BRAIN as their first product—and it's the one nootropic supplement I found that fit my criteria for This Stuff. That is, it's not banned by WADA, so athletes can use it; athletes actually do use it (or at least endorse it); and—this is the biggie—scientific studies have found that it actually seems to work.

Onnit founder Aubrey Marcus tells me that he was an athlete in high school—a basketball player, mainly—and that his mother, a nutritional doctor, was always giving him different supplements. He also tells me he started Onnit and created Alpha BRAIN because he was frustrated by the supplement landscape. He seems most passionate about this, saying, "The supplement industry generally falls into two categories. One is the natural ingredients, but you don't ever feel them. The other is that they're chemical-based ingredients, and you do feel something, but you have to pay the taxes on the back end."

They may well make you feel like crap and get you sick.

Marcus says he didn't believe those were the only options. He wanted to find the golden egg of supplements: natural, powerful, and scientifically valid. He says, "Right now I don't know of another supplement with the kind of natural ingredients that we use that also has the same rigor of clinical validation that Alpha BRAIN has."

For what it's worth, I couldn't find anything either.

The ingredients include *Bacopa monnieri*, cat's claw, *Huperzia serrata* extract, and oat straw.

Bacopa monnieri comes from a flower found in India, used by Indian physicians to improve memory and longevity. It can be both an antioxidant and an adaptogenic. *Adaptogenic* means the flower contains *adaptogens,* known to stabilize some of our physiological processes and promote that homeostasis that Pierre Beauchamp taught me about, the holiest of holy grails for the human body.

Cat's claw—found in the Amazonian rain forest—is a plant known for being rich in antioxidants and for boosting the human immune system.

Huperzia serrata extract comes from a plant that promotes the creation of the neurotransmitter acetylcholine, which is critical for muscle function and neuron communication.

Finally, oat straw—scientific name *Avena sativa*—eases stress and staves off exhaustion; EEG tests have shown oat straw to enhance alpha-brain-wave dominance.

I tried both the Alpha BRAIN pills, which are pretty standard-sized capsules and go down easy, and Alpha BRAIN Instant, a powder that mixes with water or Gatorade or whatever. It tastes good. Just about every time I tried the pills or the powder—a couple dozen times each, at least—I felt good. Alert. Focused. It feels like coffee, except without the jitters and then crash, giving me a mellow sort of energy.

Some caveats: when Marcus first launched Onnit, it was solely a supplement company, and Internet sleuths caught him pulling the age-old supplement marketing trick of massaging scientific claims in less-than-factual ways and using marketing jargon full of life-changing promises. Now Onnit, which has expanded beyond supplements into food, fitness equipment, and clothing, comes off as far less jargony and more grounded.

One of Onnit's business partners is Joe Rogan, the comedian, UFC analyst, and host of *The Joe Rogan Experience,* a popular podcast downloaded millions of times every month. Both Rogan and the Onnit people say that what drives them is simply a desire to make cool stuff that helps them, and then help other people find it. And along the way, they've built a $28 million business.

All that said, regardless of what Marcus's methods were before, and regardless of people's opinion of him—and wow, do people on the Internet have opinions of him—nothing matters in the face of science. Alpha BRAIN is in the early stages of scientific testing, and so far the results are worth a look.

The first Alpha BRAIN study was published in 2014 and conducted by neuropsychologists and neurologists at the Memory Clinic in Bennington, Vermont, the Boston Center for Memory, the Boston University School of Medicine, and Williams College in Williamston, Massachusetts. They took seventeen people between eighteen and thirty-five years old and randomly chose about half of them to take Alpha BRAIN. Then, all seventeen underwent "a comprehensive battery of neuropsychological tests," after which they "followed manufacturer's instructions for use of Alpha BRAIN for six weeks."

Six weeks later, they were all tested again. The control group—

which didn't get Alpha BRAIN—scored about the same as they did the first time. The Alpha BRAIN group, however, showed "significant improvement on several outcome measures."

The next study came a year later, conducted by the same group. This one nearly quadrupled the number of participants and used the same process. It replicated the results of the first: once again, Alpha BRAIN helped participants, on average by 12 percent, at verbal recall and 21 percent on an executive function test. In addition, participants reported that Alpha BRAIN caused no adverse side effects.

This study also used EEG assessments, which found that the brain waves of folks taking Alpha BRAIN generated much stronger alpha waves, with lower theta-beta ratios, meaning they were more relaxed and focused.

ADDICTION

A final note on the subject of drugs: some fascinating research has come up in the world of addiction. Our understanding of the subject is still evolving, but according to Maia Szalavitz, a junkie-turned-neuroscientist and the author of *Unbroken Brain,* one thing is clear: in a June 2016 article for the *New York Times,* she wrote that she's come to see addiction not as a disease, nor some sort of sin, but as a learning disorder. The brain compels the addict in unique ways, and that compulsion can, she writes, be redirected with proper care: "This type of wiring can be a benefit, not just a disability . . . The ability to persevere is an asset: People with addiction just need to learn how to redirect it."

Sound familiar? This echoes Mike Gervais and Urban Meyer describing "disorders" as potential gifts, capable of growing into something like superpowers.

That said, no matter who uses drugs, the general effects remain the same: the drug will change Big Fronty, arguably the most important part of being a human being, as it governs motivation, inhibitory control, and choice.

Drugs also alter the brain's *basolateral amygdala*—part of Migsby—which is believed to link emotion with an event, location, or some other sort of stimulus. You know those fun beer commercials? You know why they make them so fun? So you associate beer with fun. Explaining this to a neuroscience journal recently, Dr. David Belin gave the example of choosing between eating cake or an apple: "[Migsby] stores the pleasurable memories associated with eating the cake, but [Big Fronty] manipulates this information, helping you to weigh up whether or not you should eat another slice or choose the apple instead. If you eat the slice, regions of the *ventral striatum,* the structure that processes reward and links emotions to actions, are activated."

On top of that, Dr. Belin and his colleague Dr. Barry Everitt conducted new research that showed *other* neuronal circuits driving drug users to seek more drugs: they come from the fear system, namely Migsby, and part of Migsby is linked to the *dorsolateral striatum,* known as "the neural locus" for habits—that is, a primary place where habits live in the brain. These pathways become so difficult to reroute because oftentimes we aren't even conscious that they are doing anything—they don't route through Big Fronty, meaning that even though they drive *urges* that lead to *thoughts* that lead to *behaviors,* we are not conscious participants in that process.

In other words, as Belin explained, when addicts go looking for a fix, they're likely not making a conscious choice to do so. Not to say they are unaware, in some sort of fugue state—they can even be trying to stop themselves, and yet feel rendered powerless. "It's a shortcut, or back door, directly to habit," Belin said. "It means that addicts can have internal urges that they are not aware of that drive drug seeking."

This is how someone who's been sober for five years can suddenly go into a full-blown relapse without realizing it. As Belin puts it, they'll tell a counselor, "I was walking down the street, and I found myself with a glass of wine, and I promise you, I didn't want it." Belin said, "This has often been dismissed as a 'weakness of the will' and then denial." That happens sometimes, too, of course, but Belin said that his research on rats shows that sometimes in certain brains, the parts responsible for motivation will link straight up with the habit parts of the brain without the person having a clue that it's happening.

This discovery was a major breakthrough.

We can get addicted to anything, but drugs' notorious reputation for consuming someone's life makes plenty of people uncomfortable with them, and not wrongly so. To quote the great comedian Louis C.K., "Drugs are so good they'll ruin your life."

Believe it or not, This Stuff has a solution for that, too: the rise of wearable technology that promises athletes the effects of a drug . . . without the drug.

Chapter 10

Shocking Potential

Plenty of athletes prefer to avoid drugs and the supplement industry altogether, but still want the same effects. This has given rise to something its makers claim can replace the aforementioned drugs completely, a cutting-edge piece of wearable tech that is sci-fi as all heck, promising to send you into a state of either unstoppable drive and focus, or utter calm and relaxation, simply by sticking it onto your head and then letting it electrocute you into your desired state of being. Your regular workouts become super workouts, and you can push your body beyond what you once thought were its limits, all by putting on a set of headphones.

Athletes are literally shocking their brains using techniques called "transcranial direct-current stimulation" (tDCS) and "transcutaneous electrical nerve stimulation" (TENS).

This is an old concept, in a way. To treat headaches, the ancient Romans would take electric eels and slap them upside people's heads.

Now scientists and businessmen and women are collaborating to create wearable devices that use electricity to help them in nearly every phase of performance, from getting them amped up and ready to play their best before a game to relaxing them afterward so that they can recover and get a good night's rest, and even electrifying their brain *during* workouts.

THYNC

One day in February 2016, Josh Norman, the All-Pro NFL cornerback who rose to prominence with the Carolina Panthers and now plays for the Washington Redskins, posted an odd picture to Facebook. He had a triangular-ish, curved white slice of plastic the length of an index finger seemingly stuck to his forehead above his right eyebrow, and he captioned the pic, simply, "#VIBINNNNN!!!"

That device is called Thync, and it is filled with technology that promises to replace your coffee and wine by—literally—electrifying you. The Thync.com website says it was created by "a team of neurobiologists, neuroscientists, and consumer electronic specialists from institutions including MIT, Stanford, [and] Harvard who are experts in our fields. We decided to put our brains together and see if there was a way to tap into our full potential without the use of chemical supplements."

They've gone about this by creating what they call "vibes"—either "Calm" or "Energy" vibes—which they describe as "neuro-signaling technology" that they say "builds upon the best features of long-standing tDCS and TENS techniques."

The way Thync works is by using the "vibe" strips—either Energy or Calm—to send currents of electricity, up to twenty milliamps strong, into the nerves on the skin of your forehead, where you place the Thync device, either behind your ear (Energy), or on the back of your neck (Calm). Once the Thync device is charged, you connect it to your phone via Bluetooth. You also have to download the Thync app. Through this app you control the type of Vibe you want, and how intense it is, and how long it lasts.

Thync's marketing team sells this with the idea that these vibes tap into the body's nervous system, activating either the sympathetic (Energy) or parasympathetic (Calm) nervous system. They claim that the Energy vibes activate your "adrenaline system," while the Calm vibes "slow down the production of stress." In short, what they do is either increase or decrease the amount of norepinephrine your brain produces.

This raises questions about whether wearables like Thync should even be legal for athletes. For now, WADA only bans drugs—and besides, even if they did ban such tech, there's no way to test for it.

All that said, I've been able to find a grand total of *two* athletes who use Thync: Norman, and world-record-holding ultrarunner Dean Karnazes, whose achievements include running fifty marathons in fifty days and once running 350 miles over eighty-two straight hours.

Norman says Thync helps him calm down after games. In July 2016, he told *Business Insider* that he was introduced to Thync at Super Bowl 50 (so, right before the February Facebook post), but he planned to use it more moving forward. "I get so high and intense," he said. Thync, he added, makes it, "So I don't have to use any pills to calm me down . . . It's part of a clean lifestyle." He said that when he uses it, within five minutes, "You're just in this state of calmness."

As for Karnazes, he's told *Sports Illustrated* that he'd use Thync's Energy vibes for a jolt out the door in the morning—

echoing the Thync marketing department's "replace your coffee" talking point—but that the Calm vibes are his favorite, helping him sleep. The Thync Calm vibe effect purports to mimic beta-blockers, which are banned by WADA—they lower the heart rate, reduce tremors, and ease anxiety by blocking the brain's norepinephrine receptors. Thync's Calm vibe, in contrast, reduces the amount of norepinephrine the body produces, creating a similar effect.

Karnazes says the product helps him sleep, which Thync really plays up on their website, making the leap between Karnazes's restful Thync-induced sleep and his ability to train harder and recover faster. Problem is, Karnazes is a freak of nature, and I mean that in the kindest, most admiring way: he doesn't *have* to recover the same way as most athletes. Most of us have a *lactate threshold*. Exert the body beyond your threshold, and you start to feel that burning in the muscles, and then you get tired and start breathing hard and all that. The lactate threshold comes from the by-product of glucose you break down when, say, running. The body can use this lactate as fuel in addition to the glucose, but when your body can't convert it to fuel faster than you produce it, you've reached your threshold.

Karnazes doesn't seem to have a lactate threshold. Like, at all. The *Guardian* once wrote that he "seems as if he can run forever," and reports that Karnazes has never so much as suffered a single muscle cramp, even running hundreds of miles at a time. He told the *Guardian*, "No matter how hard I push, my muscles never seize up. That's kind of a nice thing if I plan to run a long way."

Karnazes's biggest problem is running until he gets sleepy. He's actually fallen asleep while running.

So while Thync might help Karnazes sleep, it's impossible to say how much it actually helps him recover, and Thync's claim that it helps him recover faster is marketing-speak at its finest.

When I first came across Thync, I was fired *up*. Probably too excited. (I'm prone to such overexcitement.) I'd *love* for "neurosignaling," as Thync calls it, to make me my most productive, calm, best self "without the use of chemical supplements."

And that said, now I'm skeptical. I got a Thync device. Tried it a lot. And I kind of hated it. The Energy vibes mostly made me irritable and edgy. The Calm vibes were better. Sometimes they didn't do much of anything, but sometimes, yeah, I felt sleepy. Not quite the "lit" high that some folks describe getting from it online, but sleepy, sure.

But again, remember the placebo effect. A lot of times, simply knowing that you're doing something will make you feel better.

The Thync folks tell you to experiment until you find what works for you, but I never found a good setting. Every once in a while the Energy vibes left me feeling clearheaded and ready to work, but the effect wasn't consistent, and mostly it left me feeling uneven. Basically, I never knew what to expect from the device, and didn't feel like I had enough control of it to get what I really needed out of it, so I got pretty tired of it pretty quickly.

As I looked more into the science that Thync offers as proof of its efficacy, the company seemed to be pulling the same sort of marketing misdirection that afflicts the chemical supplement industry. Their website says that they've done scientific studies that prove ten-minute vibes every day for a week reduce stress and improve mood, but when I ask about those studies, they just send me a link to a page on their website with *lots* of scientific papers about the methodology in *general*, but not about Thync specifically. This is a common bit of misdirection among supplement companies.

In any event, the closest thing I could find to a real-world scientific examination came when I stumbled across a video at

GQ's website featuring tech writer Brent Rose. He found that using Thync's Energy vibes made him type faster and more accurately and drive faster around a go-kart track, and that its Calm vibes helped him calm down after unexpected Taserings—he had a buddy flip a coin and then either Taser him or not, without warning—and before a Tinder date. Which he had professionally filmed and documented, by the way. By the end of the evening, he even got his date in on the action and they vibed out together. Of course, this was also after a few adult beverages, including, in Rose's words, "a bowl of beer."

In any event, they ended the date with a toast to painful experiences. "And by that," Rose said jubilantly, "I mean this whole date."

And then the girl kissed him.

Lovely as that was, it still didn't give me a good scientific answer.

So I called Dr. Greg Appelbaum, a neuroscientist at Duke. He's an expert in all kinds of stuff, including electric stim. He's done a lot of experiments and studies at Duke, including one on whether electric stim can help surgeons in the operating room. When it comes to the kind of "neurosignaling" that Thync is talking about, Appelbaum is skeptical at best. For now, he says, "Electrical stimulation for improving sports performance is probably closer to snake oil than science."

That cast a bit of a shadow on this *other* electric stim device I found, called Halo Sport, a set of headphones that claims to "help athletes train 50 percent faster."

HALO SPORT

If you watched the U.S. Olympic ski-jumping team train in 2015, you saw them wearing big, bulky, over-the-ear headphones. The headphones' headband dug into their skulls with rows and rows of little silicone teeth. That headset is the Halo Sport, which sends electricity through the skin and skull and brain, and into the *motor cortex*, which it is activating in order to ensure that the athletes leave no extra energy on the table come time to, say, jump off a ski ramp.

Or at least that's the sales pitch from Dr. Daniel Chao, the inventor.

The skiers aren't alone. Chao's gotten Halo a lot of press recently, not the least of which came in March 2016, when the device was linked directly to the most dominant team in the NBA that season, the Golden State Warriors. Forward James McAdoo tweeted out a picture of himself working out wearing the Halo headphones and thanking Halo for letting him and his teammates use them. (Neither Chao, anyone at Halo, nor anyone on the Warriors would comment further about that, except to say that yeah, a bunch of the Warriors' players have been using them.)

By all appearances, Chao's onto something. According to his in-house case study, after training with Halo Sport for four weeks, Olympic ski jumpers increased their propulsive force by 13 percent.

Not only does the motor cortex act as mission control for the muscles, orchestrating contractions and coordinated movements throughout the body, but it also serves as the muscles' battery. Muscles require electric stimulation to do their muscle things; the motor cortex powers said muscular electricity. Broadly speaking, it is responsible for both skill *and* strength.

Using something to send electricity through the skull and into the motor cortex, Chao says, temporarily puts it into a state of "hyperplasticity." When part of the brain becomes hyperplastic, it's easier to influence with training. With Halo Sport, the idea is to stimulate the motor cortex into said hyperplastic state, then go work out, thus realizing more gains than the athletes would without Halo.

Halo uses tDCS, and the medical tDCS technique has definitely been proven to work. The way tDCS operates is surprisingly simple: stick two electrodes on opposite sides of your head and connect them to some source of electricity. You *could* use a nine-volt battery if you want (not recommended). Where the electrodes are placed guides the current. One sends, the other receives the electricity rippling through the brain from one to the other. This current sparks the neurons to send more go signals or slow signals, depending on which direction it flows.

At least two thousand tDCS studies have been published over the past six years, exploring everything from helping people learn, beat addiction, wade out of depression, and in Parkinson's patients, even walk better.

Researchers have even studied whether tDCS can help athletes. In 2007, a team of Italian scientists, led by neurologist Dr. Filippo Cogiamanian, found that sending electricity into the motor cortex indeed reduced fatigue and increased endurance. In 2013, a study in Brazil led by biological engineer Alexandre Okano and published in the *British Journal of Sports Medicine,* found that cyclists, after twenty minutes of tDCS, pedaled with 4 percent more power, had a lower heart rate, and felt lower perceived effort. This woke the sports world up to tDCS.

The following year, Andy Walshe at Red Bull commissioned Australian neuroscientists Dylan Edwards and David Putrino, who work at the Burke Rehabilitation Center and Weill Cornell Medical Center in New York, to create a five-day testing protocol using all kinds of brain stim—electric, magnetic, peripheral nerve stimulation, EMG, EEG, and many other tools. Walshe called it Project Endurance, and the idea was to push athletes to their breaking point, over and over again, to find what it is in the brain that makes us stop even when we seem to have more left in the tank.

The athletes they tested include six-time cyclocross national champion Tim Johnson, mountain biker Rebecca Rusch, and BMX rider Mike Day, along with triathletes Jesse Thomas and Sarah Piampiano. Thomas, later writing about it for the *Red Bulletin*, said, "Physically and mentally, this was one of the most stressful training experiences I've ever had."

Rusch was the first to get on a bike in the lab—and thus the first to get all strapped in, which included, among other physiological monitors, a neoprene cap similar to the one Dr. Dan Chartier used for my EEG assessment, with eight electrodes on it. One sent the tDCS current, another received it, and the remaining six acted as an EEG monitor. After twenty minutes of treatment, the athletes rode their stationary bikes while undergoing a series of brutal in-lab endurance tests. In order to see how the tDCS was working—or if it was at all—the doctors gave some athletes real tDCS treatments, others a fake treatment, and none of them knew what they were getting.

"My first thought," Rusch said, "was, 'How is this different from the electroshock therapy they did in the fifties?'"

The difference is that electroshock therapy hit those patients with five hundred to a thousand times more current, strong enough to cause a seizure.

Rusch wanted in because, as she told the cluster of scientists and a small group of journalists, she wanted to know how to tap into something more. "If you're being chased by a lion," she says, "or a car falls on a baby, you find something extra. I think we're just touching the iceberg of 'How do we train that?'"

After, in Thomas's words, "three days of brutality" in the lab, the athletes and crew went to the StubHub velodrome—a cycle-racing track—in Carson, California, for some electric stim and four-kilometer time trials.

During the first, Johnson was the fastest, at 5:20, beating Thomas by two seconds.

A few hours and another brain stim treatment later, they went again, and this time Thomas shaved twelve seconds off his time, down to 5:10, while Johnson did well but still finished seven seconds behind Thomas, at 5:17.

Now, whether the tDCS helped them . . . that's hard to say. Short answer is, not really: during the first trial, which Johnson won, the real treatment went to Thomas, while Johnson got a fake treatment.

The second trial, which Thomas won—and during which he shaved off those twelve seconds—he actually received a fake treatment, while Johnson got the real thing.

"You can do all this shit," Johnson said, "but it all comes down to two guys on a bike, trying to beat each other."

Andy Walshe has since become an adviser to Halo, and he loves their concept and is encouraged by their early research. Those ski-jumper numbers aren't nothing. "They're letting the data speak for itself," he says. "Which is all you can do."

And Chao does. I spent a good while on the phone with him, and he seemed earnest and sincere about wanting to create something legitimately useful. After graduating from Stanford's medical school, Chao says, his entire professional life has been about the brain, and he says he came up with the idea for Halo after years of working as a medical doctor.

Halo is actually his second brain-stimulation company; Neuro-Pace was the first, where he helped build, essentially, a pacemaker for the brain that helped epilepsy patients. Chao says he and his colleagues created "the world's first closed-loop neurostimulator," meaning the device handles everything from identifying problems to fixing them. The device, called the RNS System, monitors the brain's electric signals, and, when detecting irregularities that can lead to seizure, is smart enough and well equipped enough to then do something about it, delivering a little electrical impulse that evens things out. All of that got packed into a tiny pulse generator the size of a small matchbox, which surgeons implant in the brain itself. Has its own battery, computer chip, software, hardware.

Today, the RNS System is available at most of the one-hundred-fifty-plus Comprehensive Epilepsy Centers in the United States.

While working at NeuroPace, Chao started wondering if something similar could be done for athletes to make them better while also, you know, *not* cutting their skull open and sticking something in their brain. Surely, he figured, scientists *had* to be capable of more with neurostimulation without surgery. "I'd always been interested in ways to stimulate the brain that could be done from the outside," he says. Putting it frankly, he says, "I believed the industry had gotten lazy."

Around 2007, Chao came across a paper by German neuroscientist Michael Nitsche that described how Nitsche activated neurons precisely the way Chao hoped was possible: stimulating them from outside the skull. He says, "It was like a new technology was discovered."

Chao kept tabs on Nitsche's work, and kept seeing more labs and scientists picking up on it and getting results over the years. Once NeuroPace was in good shape, Chao felt like he had to try building something himself. He convinced his friend and NeuroPace colleague Brett Wingeier to join him, and in 2013, they both quit their jobs and went to work.

Although Chao had been thinking about athletes, sports weren't his first goal—he just wanted to build something that could do what Nitsche and the rest had said was possible, only better and more accessible for the everyman. But as they worked,

Chao says they tested more than a thousand people before deciding to focus on creating a device targeting the motor cortex. Once they decided to start there, next came the obvious question: "Who the heck would want this?" Chao says. "And that led us to elite athletes."

And as Walshe says, Chao is certainly letting the data speak for itself, saying, "This technology is real. I've seen the data. There's no doubt in my mind we're getting results with this thing." The only thing that makes me itchy about Chao is what he doesn't say, which is something he *surely* must know after all his years working in the medical field: the problem is, there's no question that the results *could* be because of Halo, but it could also be the placebo effect.

Because here's something else Chao has to know: as much research as there is out there showing that tDCS works, other studies have shown that it might not work at all, at least not the way Chao's describing. In April 2016, New York University's György Buzsáki presented a study wherein he found that, of all electricity applied to the skull, only 10 percent makes it to the brain. In other words, of the twenty milliamps of electricity Halo purports to send into the motor cortex, maybe only two of those milliamps even make it. This makes critics question the effectiveness of tDCS—these results inspired one tDCS researcher to describe the entire field as "a sea of bullshit and bad science."

A couple of months later, a study presented in June 2016 at a meeting of the American College of Sports Medicine in Boston showed that tDCS did nothing for people in an intermittent sprint test, which is the sort of thing that applies neatly to, say, the Golden State Warriors and other basketball players.

I kind of hate how skeptical I feel about Halo. It's such a cool concept—*and* some of the best athletes in the world say it makes them better. That's not nothing. On top of all that, I'll just say it—I like Chao. We talked for a long time on the phone and had a good, honest, even sometimes deep conversation about all things mind and sport, not just Halo.

And yet, skepticism.

I asked Dr. Greg Appelbaum at Duke about Halo, too, hoping he could change my mind. He's a generally positive guy who loves kicking around fun new ideas. But even with all his exuberance, Appelbaum confirmed my concerns. He says in flat, certain terms, "I can't imagine that it actually works."

He explains, "The issue is that you have to target (i.e., hyperpolarize) one motor cortex at a time, and therefore can only apply it to one side of the body at a time. Unless these athletes are training one side of the body at a time (keeping in mind that the other side is probably actually impaired because it is getting depolarized) then I can't see how they can do the targeting. I could be wrong, but I doubt this is actually useful for sports training. There are two hemispheres. Each has a motor area that connects to the contralateral side of the body. Hyperpolarizing both at the same time is difficult, because you would need to place the cathodal electrode (the negative one) very far away from the anodal electrode (the positive one). That would mean either a very strong current that would hurt, or a very weak one that didn't do much."

Then what about these ski jumpers?

"I don't doubt that legitimate athletes believe that things like this work," Appelbaum says. "Simply believing that something works can have an influence."

That said, Appelbaum is intrigued. "If you can show me well-done, controlled experiments," he says, "then I might change my mind."

However, just because the effects might be placebo is not

necessarily a negative, at least in terms of helping athletes get better. David T. Martin, the director of performance research and development for the Philadelphia 76ers, worked at the Australian Institute of Sport for two decades before taking the Philly job. In 2013, he wrote an editorial for the *International Journal of Sports Physiology and Performance* that argued that sports scientists, instead of always blasting placebo effects, should maybe focus on leveraging, in his words, "belief effects."

He might not be wrong. For one thing, as he points out in his piece, stuff like caffeine, Gatorade, and blood buffers *have* been found to improve athletic performance by 1 to 3 percent—but combining them doesn't lead to some sort of exponential multiplying of improvement. Instead, benefits stay around 1 to 3 percent, which seems to indicate that we can't just layer one thing on top of another on top of another to turn the athlete into some kind of superhero. And from there, the logic says these things must be helping the athlete improve by affecting the same, single part of the body: the brain.

That, and not necessarily the electrical currents themselves, could be why Halo generates results. In April 2015, *New Yorker* science journalist Elif Batuman wrote, "tDCS may not merely trigger the placebo effect, as all treatments do, but actually amplify it."

So, is "neurosignaling" going to take over the world tomorrow? Tough to say. The concept still has a lot to prove. Right now it seems like more of a fringe component of the revolution that is This Stuff, the sort of thing that could be huge someday, or it could be a total dud and go down in venture capitalist flames.

If Thync and Halo do fail, though, someone somewhere may

still come up with a valid product that does all the great things they first set out to do.

And in that way, like much of This Stuff, although this may not be *the* future, it gives us a sign that the future is bright and full of promise.

Chapter 11

A Delightful Hijacking

While the neurosignaling promises of Thync and Halo might ring somewhat hollow, there is something else, NuCalm, that also uses electric stim, though as one part of a larger system designed to thrust someone into a deep state of what could be described as forced meditation . . . on steroids.

The NuCalm system consists of a protein supplement, electric stim, light-blocking eye mask, and noise-canceling headphones playing proprietary "neuroacoustic" software. It was first introduced to the world of sports about five years ago, in a back room at a dentist's office just outside of Chicago.

In the summer of 2012, sitting in a room at the offices of periodontist Dr. Paul J. Denemark, Chicago Blackhawks head trainer Mike Gapski was getting on David Poole's nerves.

Poole was *trying* to tell Gapski about NuCalm. Gapski called him a couple days earlier asking all kinds of questions about Nu-

Calm after Denemark told Gapski he should consider using it on his hockey players (Denemark used it on his dental-phobic patients with almost perfect success). But now that they were in the room together, Gapski kept huffing and grunting nonreplies and glancing at his watch, like he had a million better places to be.

Gee, sorry to waste your time, Poole thought.

Finally Poole said to Gapski, "You know what, talk is cheap. Let's just do it. You have time?"

Eh, yeah, guess so.

"I won't keep you long—no longer than you want to stay."

Gapski said all right, and Poole set him up. *Sit in this chair, get comfy. Take this cream, it's a protein supplement thing, I'll explain later, just rub it up and down each carotid artery, yep. Now these are neurostimulation patches, stick them behind your ears. This thing I'm plugging them into, that's a cranial electric-stimulation device. Don't worry, we use so little power—like, 0.1 milliamps— that you won't even feel it on your skin. Now take this eye mask, get it around your head. Now put these headphones on, they're wireless, over the ear, block out all sound, and they'll play our—well, we'll talk about that later, too. If you want. If you have the time. Okay, all set? Music on? Now just pop on that eye mask and let me know when you're ready to quit. Whenever you're out of time.*

Ten minutes went by.

Then twenty.

Then forty. Gapski seemed unconscious. That's when Poole knew Gapski must've been really stressed. The more stressed or anxious someone is, the more strongly NuCalm affects them.

At fifty minutes, Poole tugged the earphones away and asked Gapski how he felt.

"I feel good," Gapski said, slipping off the eye mask. "Why? What's going on?"

"How long you think you've been in?"

"I don't know. Ten minutes?"

"It's been fifty-one minutes, Mike."

Gapski gave Poole a look that said, *You're crazy.* Then he looked at his watch. He stood up. "Okay. What the hell. Now you have my attention."

Poole's tone is rapid and excited as he tells me this story early last year in his thick Boston accent. "Mike was *cooked*," Poole says. "I mean, he was out to *lunch*, minutes in. He said, 'I'm a different person now. You did something to me, and I don't know what.' I said, 'Yeah, you were a total asshole an hour ago. Now you seem like a reasonable guy!'"

Poole's meeting with Gapski was a couple of months before the scheduled start of the NHL season. The Blackhawks were plenty good before NuCalm—they won the 2010 Stanley Cup—but after getting a bunch of NuCalm systems just prior to the 2012 season (which, due to a lockout, didn't end up starting until January 2013), they won the Stanley Cup that year and then again just two years later, in 2015.

In his NuCalm testimonial on the company's website, Gapski says, "You could tell that these guys were just more relaxed." He says that his goal as a trainer is to make his players "play 'intense' and not 'tense,'" and Nucalm "is a way for them to just relax and deal with frustrations." Gapski goes on to say that NuCalm clears his and his players' heads, and that it is hugely helpful with recovery, "a crucial part of this game." And, he adds, "I think NuCalm played an important role for us, especially during the playoffs."

After trying NuCalm, Gapski ordered three units, and soon after that ordered a dozen more that were shared among the players. As with all This Stuff, some guys weren't fans, but a lot loved it. Then came the playoffs, and Gapski ordered six more systems, and, Poole says, the NuCalm team was constantly having to ship the Blackhawks more supplies.

After the major grind of that compressed 2013 lockout season, Gapski saw guys wearing down more every day, their bodies just giving out. But he also saw the ones using NuCalm seeming to recover faster than the rest.

NuCalm acts as a sort of reset button for the autonomic nervous system—the system wherein the sympathetic and parasympathetic systems live, remember. Resetting the ANS helps the body recover in unexpected ways. One Blackhawk player dislocated his shoulder, and then, after doing NuCalm twice a week, told Poole he'd never felt better. "The first time I actually felt *good*," the guy said. He went on about it at length, saying he could feel his body rebuilding and healing.

Gapski told Poole, "There was no way some of these guys would've been on the ice without it."

Poole says now, "So that was really the beginning of *wow, there's something really interesting here.*"

When he was invited to the executive box one game, Poole says he was introduced as the NuCalm Guy, and one of the Blackhawks' executive staff said, "Oh my God! Every time I travel with these guys, everyone on the plane—you get on, and it used to be drinking and drugging and freaking out and playing poker, back when I was playing. Now? They all have these headsets on! And they're *sleeping*!"

"And he says, 'It's *bizarre*,'" Poole tells me, playfully overdoing it, implying that his thought is, *Yeah, okay, buddy.* (He's good at leading with the self-deprecation and then following with statements like: "He said, 'But whatever it's doing, it's *working*, because these guys are playing *lights-out*. Just won two [Stanley Cup championships] out of three years, blah blah blah blah blah.'")

Since the Blackhawks took up NuCalm, about twenty other teams from different sports have begun using it, too, plus some Olympians and other individual athletes.

Before Gapski and the Blackhawks, however, NuCalm was used primarily by dentists helping their patients deal with dental anxiety. NuCalm was invented by Dr. Blake Holloway, a neuroscientist who knows almost nothing about sports. He and Poole were on the phone recently with an NFL quarterback who's won the Super Bowl and been named league MVP and all that. The quarterback was asking Holloway and Poole some questions about what NuCalm could do for him, and Holloway mortified Poole by starting his answer to this football superstar with the words, "Okay, well, let's imagine you were a quarterback in the NFL . . ."

Long before athletes started using NuCalm to win championships, Dr. Holloway developed NuCalm while trying to find a cutting-edge way to treat PTSD and other acute mental disorders. In a company statement about NuCalm, he says, "We are currently living in the second age of anxiety, the first being just after World War I. People are more stressed today than during the Great Depression, and not doing enough to manage [it]."

PTSD resides on the furthest reaches of the darkest edge of the trauma spectrum. One would be hard-pressed to find trauma greater than severe PTSD, which leaves your body in essentially a constant state of sympathetic drive, meaning your fight-or-flight response is almost always turned on. Poole says that for the human brain, it's like trying to pump 220 volts of electricity through a conductor capable of processing only 110 volts. "If you don't explode and disappear," he says, "that energy's gotta go somewhere. And it remaps your brain terrain. It rewires your brain to a very unhealthy state. And your body is in a constant state of panic."

This is a big reason why someone with PTSD is also prone to alcoholism and drug addiction. The brain seeks out ways to cope and will use whatever seems easiest unless consciously directed otherwise.

Holloway wanted to relieve traumatized brains without drugs. EEG training *can* do this, but he wanted to come up with something easier.

It took him four years.

And now there's NuCalm. In July 2015, after several years and more than six figures' worth of research, NuCalm was awarded a patent (number 9,079,030) by the U.S. Patent and Trademark Office. This is the only patent for technology that reduces stress and improves sleep in the world. "Which is absolutely insane to me," Poole says. "It's like, shame on pharmacology. Shame on the research communities. They could solve this problem in a weekend, but they make money selling pills, even if they have more side effects than benefits."

What frustrates Holloway and Poole and others about the pharmaceutical world is its exploitation of consumers' ignorance. For instance, I had no clue, until I started this project—years after I started taking some medication to manage my struggles—that some of the medications I've taken can take a *year and a half* to work their way out of my system, and that only after I completely cut them off. In the meantime, they can clog some of the brain's synapses, which can be damaging.

Pills can be useful, even lifesaving, but they are not a cure. They can be a crucial oxygen mask in a fire, but they don't put the fire out.

NuCalm is four different therapies rolled into one. Two of those interrupt the stress response in the brain, the other two interrupt it in the body.

Part of NuCalm's goal is to disrupt the unnatural rhythm that modern society has created for our brains. When we wake up in the morning and first see the sunlight, it activates our sympathetic nervous system. That, you probably remember from earlier, floods us with adrenaline and causes us to scan our environment for threats. Problem is, modern life throws our body's natural rhythms out of whack with all of its lights, cell phones, caffeine, television screens, smartphones, and so on. We don't start getting sleepy just because the sun goes down anymore. There's always something to do and something to distract us—and there is so much artificial light in our lives now, which tells our brains to stop creating *melatonin*, which helps us relax and sleep. We've juked our natural system. Artificial light stimulates us like the sun, keeps our threat detection systems humming in the brain, and keeps the adrenaline flowing.

One thing NuCalm does is activate the brain's *GABAergic system*. There's a lot of complex chemistry and science involved; the important detail here is the GABA (*gamma-Aminobutyric acid*), which is the primary neurotransmitter responsible for sending stop signals to neurons and blocking go signals. In the context of someone with an overactive brain, then, with enough GABA, the neurons wouldn't hear *relax relax relax*, exactly, but the signals getting them all worked up would hit the brakes.

Dr. Holloway developed a supplement that delivers loads of GABA to Big Fronty. This used to come as a pill, though they are now transitioning to a cream-based delivery system applied to the skin over the carotid arteries on the neck, absorbed into the bloodstream, and then pooled with Big Fronty. That's not going to do anything for you itself, though. Your body naturally collects GABA all day from food, but that GABA doesn't kick in until the brain calms down enough, typically when we're falling asleep.

Enter NuCalm's electric stim.

Two adhesive patches go behind the ears on the soft spot between the skull and the jaw. That's a pressure point with direct access to Big Fronty. These patches connect to a cranial electric stimulation (CES) device, which delivers .1 milliamps of electric current through the patches and into the skin. That's a small amount, just enough juice to give Big Fronty's GABA receptors a nudge. Simply put, this tells them to bind with the GABA being stored up there. This sets about disrupting the brain's stress response, shutting down the production of adrenaline in the midbrain and telling your brain to start chilling out. However, this is not a particularly dramatic or predictable phase of the process, comparable, at best, to having a glass of wine—in fact, Poole says, "We're actually working on the same receptor sites in the brain that alcohol works on."

With this, the overactive sympathetic system creating irrational behavior will grind to a halt. Remember: this was all originally designed for people with PTSD, engineered to take someone ready to fight the world at all times and put them into a state of calm.

It's a good start, but still far from the deep relaxation such patients need, and does not last.

How that starts to happen is, Poole says, "the real sexy part."

That real sexy part is when NuCalm hypnotizes you at the midbrain.

The way this works is mega-trippy, in the best way. Part of the NuCalm system is a pair of headphones that come with built-in software that plays proprietary NuCalm music (they call it "neuroacoustic software") directly from the headphones themselves. At first, the music sounds like nothing more than generic classical music, but listen close, and you hear the secret stuff beneath the violins and pianos: strange pulsating tones, reminiscent of the eerie sounds we usually associate with aliens and *The X-Files*.

These tones create the phenomenon known as "binaural beats," discovered in 1839 by physicist Heinrich Wilhelm Dove. Ever since I learned about them, I listen to them as much as I do regular music.

To put it basically, binaural beats don't really exist.

They work like this: tones of two different frequency levels are played into each ear. (You have to use headphones, and the two separate tones have to be within 40 Hertz of one another or it won't work.) When your ears collect that data and present it to the midbrain, the brain doesn't know what to do with it. The brain can't process two separate frequencies like that, so instead, to make any sense out of what's going on, it just creates its own third frequency out of the difference between the two incoming tones. If your brain picks up a tone of, say, 32 Hertz from your right ear, and a tone of 24 Hertz from your left ear, it will interpret that as a tone of 8 Hertz. And that made-up third tone is the binaural beat.

If your brain hears enough of that binaural beat for a long enough time—usually no more than a few minutes—then your brain waves will follow the beat. So as the brain gets more and more of that 8 Hertz, it will eventually generate alpha-brain-wave activity long enough that your brain slips into an alpha-dominant state.

(And ditto for any binaural beat in any of the other brain-wave ranges.)

NuCalm's binaural beats are engineered to induce that low alpha state, putting you on the edge between deep relaxation and sleep. "Binaural beats brain entrainment," Poole calls it. "There's no way to detect it, and resistance is futile."

When everything is good to go—lotion on, patches on, CES electrifying you, music playing—then it's time for the final piece: a simple blackout eye mask.

In combination, it all locks the brain into a state akin to deep meditation.

And boom, there you are: "NuCalming."

Poole says that no matter what state I'm in—even super stress with high beta brain waves running wild—a few minutes of Nu-

Calm will take care of me. "We don't care what the stress is, what the context is, we don't care who you are," he says. "I don't care how big you are, how drunk you are, it doesn't matter."

In this state, Poole says, you're in "parasympathetic nervous system dominance," which is neurospeak for "you are mega chilled out." Your alpha brain waves are dominant, and you're in something of a trance, and you'll be there as long as the headphones stay on.

It's different from meditation in that you're not consciously using meditation techniques and such to put yourself into this sort of state of mind—or at least, you don't have to—but what ends up happening in the mind is similar. Instead of shutting down and going to sleep, the mind wanders freely. Anxious thoughts might come to mind—a game, a flight, a dental appointment—and your brain *will* respond. *Oh, I hear the drill, I see the needle, we're having turbulence,* whatever, but—and this is the key here—the *body* will not, in turn, generate the typical stress response I've learned so much about. The adrenal glands won't flood us with epinephrine, the heart won't race, the muscles will remain loose, the lungs will pump in full. And in this way, we're able to sort through anything upsetting without causing further damage to ourselves. And eventually, we'll be able to heal.

When, say, the Blackhawks use NuCalm before games, it leaves them in that state of mind, or much closer to it, for three or more hours. "When Jordan goes for eighty points or whatever," Poole says, "and the game comes so easy, and is so slow, he is not anxious, he is not stressed. That 'ice in the veins' phenomenon? That's the alpha state of consciousness. That's your creative, relaxed zone. That's your automatic zone. You want things to be intuitive—you don't want to be reacting to things and thinking about them."

And after the game, NuCalm can help someone calm down—it

promotes natural breathing that helps with sleep, too, akin to what Pierre Beauchamp and the Mindroom crew were teaching me.

NuCalm, by the meditative state it induces, also creates relaxation by helping athletes separate analysis of a problem from the emotion of it. In other words, when settled into a NuCalm session, the athlete can think about ways to improve without arousing the emotion associated with bad memories. Poole and Holloway use Tiger Woods as an example of an athlete who has seemed unable to do this. After blowing up his marriage, one of the changes Woods made was to reconstruct his golf swing. Holloway called Poole and said, "You know I don't know anything about sports, right?"

"Yeah," Poole said, remembering the quarterback conversation. "I am aware of that."

"I'll tell you right now, Tiger Woods will never win another championship. You do not destroy the muscle memory. You move *on* from a bad event. Do not deconstruct what you've done ten thousand times."

Poole says, "And sure enough, look at him now. He's awful. And that was Blake saying that once something becomes automatic, reconditioning it is really difficult, and it's not even necessary."

What's necessary is training the mind to go, *Hey, just forget it.* Missed a foul shot to lose a game, bombed in the Masters, threw four interceptions in the Super Bowl? Work harder at practice if you want to, but, Poole says, "It's all about relaxing instead of thinking about it and stressing about it. Saying, *Okay, guys, I missed that shot. I got your back tomorrow.*"

And for all the mental and psychological benefits of NuCalm, it helps your body heal same as meditation does—Poole calls the NuCalm state the "optimum healing state"—and it makes you smarter, at least temporarily. "You're getting optimal oxygenation into your blood flow to the brain," he says. "We're gonna engorge your prefrontal cortex and frontal cortex, so [they are] going to recruit more communication paths. So you're gonna be brighter, smarter, more focused for about three hours after NuCalm. Every single time you'll use it."

Poole adds that with a simple tweak to the music, they could use the system to put someone into a deep and dreamless sleep—the 0.5 to 4 Hz range—and they could just as easily make someone nightmarishly anxious. "For the Yankees, for example," he says. "I'm a Red Sox fan. If I could change the algorithm, and get the NuCalm to the Yankees, I'd put them in 45 Hertz, and they'd have diarrhea and they'd break out in rashes before every game."

Poole sends me one of their older, discontinued packages to try for my research. In the delivery box, there's a small black backpack, the NuCalm logo on the front. Inside: headphones, supplement cream, eye masks, neuropatches, CES device.

I call Poole and he walks me through the setup. He recommends giving myself an hour per session, from setup to conclusion. He ends our conversation by saying, "Have fun. You're in for a wild ride."

I'm feeling an uncomfortable mix of excitement and extreme cynicism—no *way* this thing really does all that Poole says it does. I'm not thrilled about carving an hour out of my day for it. I figure I'll give it fifteen, twenty minutes, see what it's all about, then try it some more later, when I have more time.

Plus, getting set up the first time is weird, what with the supplement cream and the "neuropatches" and the music and all that. When I'm finally good to go, I settle into a comfy chair and pull on the mask.

I'm feeling some light tingling on my neck, where the patches are, and I'm feeling edgy and anxious because I feel like I have a million other things to do, but I figure I should at least get some good notes, and maybe I'll be able to use them to better under-

stand how NuCalm might help the Blackhawks and other athletes, but then I'll need to follow up with—

Whoa.

My muscles start twitching in light little flicks, like when I'm
falling asleep. My anxiety's gone. I can think about all the things I
need to think about without all the usual stress—and wow, I didn't
realize how stressed I normally *was* over such *simple* thoughts in
the first place. It feels like meditation but better (although maybe
I'm just not very good at meditating) because I don't really have
to work that hard for it—I feel like I've climbed into a car and had
someone drive me to Meditation Land.

I never go to sleep, but I am *gone.* Cooked. Out-to-lunched.
Gapskied.

After about twenty minutes, I want to stay in longer, but there's
stuff to do, so I pull off the mask and headphones and patches,
and pull my phone out of my pocket, and—wait a minute.

It hasn't been twenty minutes. It's been over an hour.

And yeah, I feel like a new guy. I'm not saying that lightly. I
like a lot of This Stuff, but the impact of NuCalm feels more profound than most of it.

When I sit down to work afterward, I don't obsess over every problem or every sentence I need to write. I just . . . write. I
mean, I can do that sometimes, but usually writing feels frenetic
and chaotic and out of control. Not now, though.

For the rest of the day, both working and then later, hanging
out with my wife and kid, I feel calm. At peace.

Free.

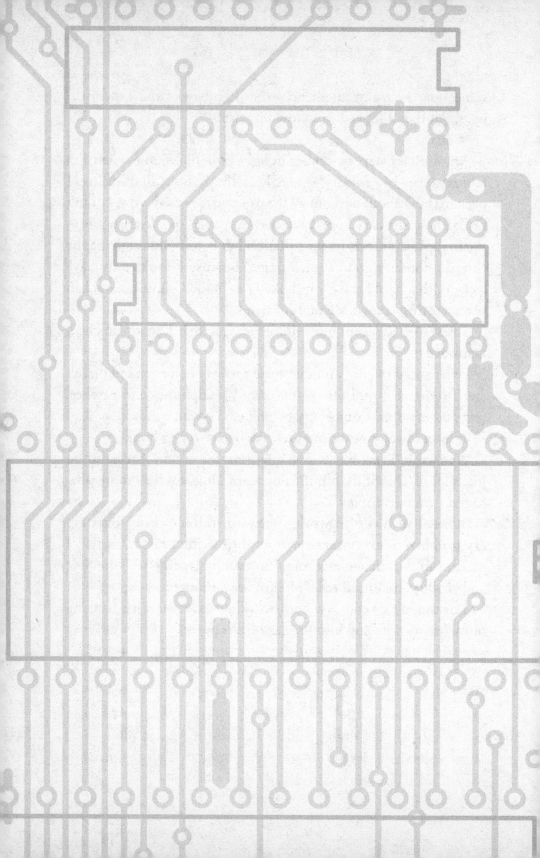

PART THREE

THE CRAFT

As I write this, the Golden State Warriors just lost the 2016 NBA Finals to the Cleveland Cavaliers after being up on them three games to one. The Cavs have done what's never been done before, and LeBron James has brought a long-craved championship to his adopted hometown. From a narrative standpoint, this is all rather beautiful. The season has been all about Steph Curry, the Warriors' dynamic, unstoppable point guard, and his apparent usurpation of King James's throne as the best basketball player in the world.

And why not? Curry became the first player in league history to be named MVP by unanimous vote. He had a monstrous season. He led the Warriors to the best record in NBA history, 73–9, besting even Michael Jordan's once-thought-un-best-able 1995–1996 Chicago Bulls. He made 402 three-pointers this season, which was 116 *more* than the standing record of 286, which *he set himself* the season before—in which, by the way, he was *also* named league MVP, and the Warriors were NBA champions. On top of that, Curry became one of the league's best all-around point guards, averaging about two steals and seven assists per game.

What I'm saying is, Curry played like some sort of alien beamed down by God for our basketball entertainment.

But then Curry hurt his knee, played kind of miserably in the 2016 finals, and, even if he *had* been healthy, who knows if he could have done anything about LeBron. After his Cavs went down 3–1, LeBron went on some sort of basketball jihad against all things Not Him Winning. LeBron was not only finals MVP, he was the first player in NBA history to lead *both* teams in five different statistical categories: points (29.7), rebounds (11.3), assists (8.9), blocks (2.3), *and* steals (2.6). It was a performance like few anyone had ever seen, and may well ever seen again, in professional basketball.

But I can't help but step back and look at Curry's story, the original narrative. That he was even there is nothing short of astonishing.

For one thing, in the Western Conference finals, he and the Warriors themselves were down 3–1 against a suddenly electrifying Oklahoma City Thunder team, and they themselves had a historic comeback. Curry was inspiring as all heck during it, culminating in the final minute of game seven, when, after a hard, scary fall to end the half—on which he made a layup—Curry was dribbling downcourt, less than a minute to play, the Warriors up six. Incredibly, the Thunder didn't foul him to stop the clock, and then Curry sprang free and drilled a three, a dagger. He turned to the crowd, smiled, and turned to his teammates and roared.

Gorgeous.

But that's not even what I mean.

What I mean is, Curry even being considered a threat to

LeBron's claim on Best in the World was unthinkable just a few short years ago. He was a kid from a little Christian school who went to Davidson College, the tiny college south of Charlotte. He carried them for a fun Cinderella run through the NCAA tournament in 2008, but NBA scouts tore him apart in their predraft scouting. One NBA scout's notes included: *Not a true point guard. Out of control at times. Limited upside. Backup/ Fringe starter. Average athleticism. Average size. Average wing- span. Frail. Relies too heavily on outside shot.* When the Warriors drafted him in 2009, at best, he seemed like he might be another Ray Allen, a great shooter, legendary even, but nothing more. Even Curry says he never dreamed his career would be so phe- nomenal. "I expected to be a pretty good NBA point guard," he once told ESPN. "And hopefully win a championship. But MVP and all this stuff? Not really. This is pretty crazy."

I mention all of this because Curry is one of the most forward- thinking athletes alive when it comes to This Stuff. Around 2011, he started working with a trainer, Brandon Payne, whose primary goal is "neurocognitive efficiency." To achieve that, they started using a lot of This Stuff. The rest is history. Literally. Curry obliterated shooting records, led the Warriors to a champion- ship (2015) and win records (seventy-three wins in 2016), and, in 2016, became the first NBA player ever to win the MVP award by unanimous vote.

Curry is even better than Payne imagined a ballplayer could be, because he is uniquely intelligent, curious, and unafraid to (a) ask questions, and (b) try new things. And man, has he tried things.

Getting the game to slow down is maybe *the* holy grail in sports. Anything you can do to make that happen, you do.

"It happens in such small quantities that you strive for it," says Jason Sada, former college soccer player and president of Axon

Sports. "And usually it's unattainable, and it happens when you don't expect it. And of course, we know that the game never really slows down. But this is what we're hearing from players. When they say 'time slows down,' that's my favorite expression, and when I was playing, that was my favorite feeling."

This is known as "time dilation prior to motor action." You are Neo in *The Matrix,* watching bullets float by you. You register complex thoughts instantly, think through everything in less time than it takes to blink. You nail the business negotiation, crush the job interview. You have an epiphany in the middle of an exhilarating discussion. You might even be psychic.

When Zack Snyder was making the movie *300,* he specifically said that he wanted to make the fight scenes look the way that sports feel to great athletes (and all great soldiers are great athletes). And those fight scenes are glorious. Snyder shows the Spartans moving rapidly toward battle, but when they are within reach of the Persians, everything goes über-slow. Then they cut them down and move on to the next, superfast—and then it's über-slow again. Rinse, repeat. Beautiful. And accurate.

This is, in part, being in the zone, in flow, on automatic, whatever you call it.

But there's more to this slowing-of-time phenomenon—and I, for one, am in awe, because it is not yet known *what* is happening in the brain when "the game slows down."

What they *do* know is that this really seems to happen. In 2012, researchers at University College London found that people *did* in fact feel time slow down before they took action. Dr. Nobuhiro Hagura of UCL's Institute of Cognitive Neuroscience said that former tennis player (and current commentator) John McEnroe "reported that he feels time slows down as he is about to hit the ball, and F1 drivers report something very similar when overtaking."

Ask any athlete who's ever been even moderately good at a sport, and they'll tell you the same thing. I felt it all the time in high school and a few times during college, when my brain wasn't turning me into a head case. It turned 90-mph fastballs into slow-pitch softballs, and, for example, when a runner tried stealing second, the bullets I could throw to get him out felt like light and simple tosses.

A popular theory among scientists is that the brain regions involved in this phenomenon include the *cerebral cortex,* the *cerebellum*, and the *basal ganglia.* Various others have put forth more theories that really get into the brain-parts weeds, including one hypothesizing that different types of sensory information—such as what you hear, see, feel, etc.—are processed at different speeds by different neural architectures.

They also think that it has to do with anticipation—which is largely the domain of the insula, the brain part that helps us predict the future. The better you predict the future, the slower it comes at you.

Hagura told the BBC, "During the motor preparation, visual information processing in the brain is enhanced. So, maybe, the amount of information coming in is increased. That makes time be perceived longer and slower . . . The brain can maximize the flow of visual input from the eyes."

The world seems to move in slow motion because the brain is working at warp speed.

"Baseball players sometimes talk about the ball looks bigger, it looks like a grapefruit," Sada says. "We know for sure the ball doesn't get bigger, right? But the brain perceives it that way. So what's happening? Well, you're probably solving problems before they've happened. The ball looks bigger because you saw it earlier and anticipated where it was going to be."

This is probably an obvious statement, but usually the only

way to get better at predicting the future is to experience all of the future's possibilities, over and over again, through practice and studying film.

Many of the folks I meet in this section bring up Malcolm Gladwell's 10,000 Hour Rule: in his book *Outliers,* Gladwell claims that it takes ten thousand hours of meaningful practice of a task to become a master. It's important to note, too, that the authors of the study he based that on say that he mistranslated the research. In spite of this, pop science writers and the like still reference the Gladwell rule pretty regularly, some of them in order to spin their own ideas about "hacking the flow state" in order to cut down the number of hours you need to master a task.

More importantly, my point here is that whether it's actually ten thousand hours, getting great at something requires endless, exhausting, repetitive, relentless physical labor. (In fact, psychologist Kevin Dutton—among others—has even wondered for the website Big Think if one needs to be a psychopath, or at least have certain psychopathic traits, to be a great athlete. That sounds absurd on its face, until Dutton lays those traits out: ruthlessness, fearlessness, mental toughness, coolness under pressure, and the ability to focus obsessively on a goal. Sounds a little too familiar, doesn't it? The key, he says, is (a) make sure there aren't any problems with aggressiveness, and (b) make sure "you're smart enough to use those superpowers for good.")

We only have so much time, and the human body can only take so much.

For instance, there's Dan McLaughlin, who in April 2010, at thirty years old, quit his job as a commercial photographer in order to put in ten thousand hours of golf and thus go pro by 2016. Problem is, his schedule got wrecked because he kept getting hurt. As of June 2016, the last update he posted to his website came on May 2, 2015, when he wrote that he was so beaten up he could only hope to chip and putt. In the update before that one, he said he still had 3,997 hours to go.

And that's only golf. Think of football drills, or swinging a bat, or kicking a soccer ball. Even if the body *could* handle ten thousand hours of those sports, it's still *so much time,* and really, that ten-thousand-hour mark Gladwell ran with might be an *un-*derestimate. Plus, it's tough to get significant time to put in the real work elite athletes need: one of the most shocking things Sada learned when he was starting his research for Axon was that, in a typical ninety-minute soccer match, a striker spends, on average, just two minutes performing on-ball decision making.

The folks discussed in this section are on a mission, each in their own way, to change that, some of them by engineering video games that pump the brain's cognitive centers like pumping biceps with weights, others by creating simulations that give athletes inconceivable amounts of practice reps, others by all of this and then some. They're not only providing athletes new ways to train in their craft, but by handing them tools that slow the game down, they are also giving them more time.

Chapter 12

The Phrase of Death

In the winter of 2011, the NBA lockout was going strong, and Steph Curry needed to work out. He drove about an hour south of his home in Charlotte, to Fort Mill, South Carolina, where he parked in front of a bland-looking warehouse. This is where Steph Curry started to become STEPH CURRY.

Inside, he worked out with Brandon Payne, the man who created and runs Accelerate Basketball, a personal coaching business. Now Curry flies Payne to Oakland all the time so they can work out; Payne spends weeks if not months on the road with him. And all of this is because, in addition to his savvy with strength training and physical conditioning, Payne is one of pro basketball's foremost experts in what he calls "neurocognitive efficiency."

Payne's goal, with Curry and with all the basketball players he works with, is to create the same amount of stress in their training environment as they will face in a game. Payne says, "Even though we're not moving them like they're in a game, even though they're not taking the punishment like they would in a game, we're training their brain in a game state of mind."

The whole idea is to prepare players for gamelike mental situations, sure, but also to help them develop and improve faster and more efficiently. That's where Payne got the name for his business in the first place: "The method and the philosophy I work off of is an accelerated program, for an accelerated rate of player development."

He and Curry are a good fit because, the way Payne puts it, "When you get into training different systems within the body, so much of it comes down to the intelligence level of the player. You have to have players who can look past the drill, who can understand the multiple layers of benefit that each drill gives them. And Steph is that kind of guy."

Payne is not only looking to work from, say, a player's toes to his fingertips in terms of shooting mechanics or skill work or strength, but, he says, "We're also working on different systems within the body to make decisions, to react quickly, to be efficient."

There are two main ways Payne goes about doing this: by creating elaborate, complex drills, and by incorporating into said drills cutting-edge tech such as strobe glasses and the FITLIGHT system. The goal is to create as much if not more stress and demand for decision-making as Curry faces in a game.

The FITLIGHT system is a bunch of palm-sized discs on poles—or just stuck on the wall, or placed on the floor—that Payne sets up during drills. It was inspired by Erik Veje Rasmussen, a handball legend in Denmark who had this idea to devise a system that could measure and train reaction time, speed, agility, and coordination. Beyond sports, FITLIGHT has partnerships with the United States military. Their goal is basic: connect what the eye sees to what the brain thinks and how the body reacts.

Payne sometimes places the FITLIGHT discs on the side as Curry goes through dribbling drills, or on the court, where Payne puts them in different spots, then controls them using a wireless remote. Each disc can be set to eight different colors, and Curry has to make certain moves and take certain shots based on what colors he sees. They'll start with two to three reads, then push up to five to six in one drill. Payne says, "It's incredibly overloading, when you've got that many decisions to make."

Their workouts shift day to day, and of course, they do much more than just train with the FITLIGHT system, but that sort of sensory overload—overwhelming the mind with stress while forcing quick decisions—is the way toward neurocognitive efficiency. Curry is being trained to adapt to high-stress, sensory-overload situations.

Say they do a seven-spot shooting drill. Curry has to make, say, eight out of ten shots at a certain spot before moving to the next. They don't count the shot as a make unless Curry not only makes the *shot,* but reads the lights correctly, too. "That's a pretty tough drill that frustrates him," Payne says. "I know when I've frustrated him, I'm doing my job, because he is not gonna stop until he beats it. And trust me, frustrating that guy is getting tougher and tougher to do."

Payne laughs when he says this, then goes on, "What people fail to realize about Stephen is that physically, in terms of his just natural maturation, [he] is just now coming into his prime. All the things we used to have to spend a lot of time on, getting stronger, and then going out on the floor, he is just naturally getting stronger now."

The reason why boils down to simple biology: Curry's physical body is simply maturing later than, say, LeBron James's did. "Some guys start to come into their physical prime when they're twenty-two, twenty-three, twenty-four," Payne says. "He's just now hitting it when he's twenty-seven. So you're going to see his rate of improvement spike. It's gonna go up tremendously for the next two years. He is just now hitting what LeBron hit when LeBron was twenty years old. Physically, he's got a lot more miles left to go and a lot of improvement left to go."

One of the main reasons I'm zooming in on Payne and Curry's work here is to highlight their core mind-set. Theirs is one that, as more people start thinking the same sort of way, is driving the greater sporting world forward—but it's also a mind-set that has met plenty of resistance.

Critics of Curry see videos of him dribbling while wearing those strobe goggles, and they hear Payne talk about neurocognitive efficiency, and they say stuff like, *All you need is a basketball and a court and a hoop,* and *All training is brain training.*

The conversations I have with Payne about this are like so many conversations I've had with so many people involved with This Stuff. He says, "Nobody's saying you can't get better that way. You certainly can. I'm just saying that the way we do it is quicker and more effective and more efficient."

Payne has been exploring different training methods for nearly twenty years. He was a solid basketball player, but short and kind of stocky, and after a couple of years playing at a Division II college, he knew he wouldn't go pro. Besides, all he'd ever wanted to be was a coach, like his dad. He quit playing when he was twenty-one, became manager of the team, and then began coaching.

As part of his first job, he managed players' skills training. That became his testing ground—he used the guys like basketball lab rats, trying one technique after another to see what helped them develop more quickly. He's also a bookworm, always hungry to learn as much as he can about how the body and the brain work, how they work together, and how he can incorporate this into his work with athletes. "The phrase of death around here in my office is, *This is just how we've always done it,*" Payne says. "Those words, I never want to hear out of anybody's mouth that works for me, because 'how we've always done it' is not as good as how we can do it today. We're smarter today than we were ten, fifteen years ago. The performance industry, and making athletes better, is still a relatively new industry. And we're learning more every day."

Even so, Payne knows his methods are sometimes a hard sell, and in some ways, his experience with them provides us with an example of what many people working on This Stuff go through. He says, "Basketball coaches, for the most part, I equate to the far radical religious right. They're so close-minded, and they want to do it the way it's always been done. Older coaches in the NBA, and even some of the younger guys, they think, *Aw, because Player X-Y-Z didn't do it back then, why do we need to do it now?* If this was available when Michael Jordan, Larry Bird, and Magic Johnson played, and we had this knowledge then, I can assure you that players that were that competitive would look for any edge they could possibly get.

"Coaches have to become more open, have to become more educated on how the body works, and the systems within the body, and how they work, in order to get their players better. Your job as a coach is to put each player in the best possible position to have success on the floor. And if you don't understand how the body works, and how that body operates while it's on the floor, you can't possibly develop that player fully.

"You can't possibly iron out all the kinks that have to be ironed out to make that player the most efficient, most injury-resistant, most skilled player he can be, because you're just doing the same things you've always done. If you tore your ACL in 1983, we put you in a cast for six months. And you were never the same after that, and we put a huge brace on your knee. After that, for the rest of your life. So, because that's how we treated it then, are we supposed to treat it the same way now? Or should we embrace the knowledge, embrace the technology, embrace the forward thinking that's occurred, and use it?"

Fifty years ago, athleticism was handled as recklessly and randomly as the mind has been handled until now. Now the world is just starting to come around to the idea that we need a certain mental fitness—as much as we need physical athleticism, we also need mental athleticism.

We'll get there. It's almost impossible to imagine now, but that's exactly how the cynics of yore talked about the physical side of sports. Fifty years ago, the fact that Boston Red Sox catcher Carl Yastrzemski spent his off-season before 1967 lifting weights with a trainer was mockable—until he hit for the Triple Crown that season. (And then, unbelievably, Yaz never lifted weights like that again, saying it was "too hard.")

Legendary Kansas City Royals infielder George Brett, who played from 1973 to 1993, told the *Hartford Courant* newspaper in 2002, "When I retired in 1993, we still didn't have a weight room. We were told to never lift weights. You'd get too muscle-bound." Then he raved about Kansas City's gigantic new cutting-edge strength and conditioning facility—complete with, he gushed, "a strength coach." He said, "We used to sit in a locker room after a game, drink beer, and eat a cheeseburger. They go in and lift now. They eat bananas. They drink all these protein drinks."

Carlton Fisk, the great catcher who played for the Boston Red Sox and the Chicago White Sox from 1969 to 1993, told the *Courant*, "When I first came up, you'd run six or eight sprints at spring training and that was supposed to get you ready for the year. You'd get fined for lifting weights or swimming."

Fisk flew in the face of that mind-set, undertaking a workout routine in the 1980s that author Doug Wilson described as "fanatical" in his 2015 biography of Fisk, *Pudge.* Fisk built a state-of-the-art weight room at his home and worked out six days a week, on four of which the workouts lasted three hours. (The other two days, ninety minutes.) Legs three days a week, upper body two, aerobics the rest. Part of his motivation was Yastrzemski himself. As a result, in 1988, at the ripe old age of forty, Fisk won the American League Silver Slugger award as the best-hitting catcher, batting .277 with nineteen home runs.

Then there's the NFL. In 1993, the *New York Times* ran an article by Thomas George highlighting these brand-new types of "strength and conditioning coaches," saying that such coaches were "finally" a normal part of the league "after years of searching for acceptance in the NFL." (That same article even had to spell out the differences between machine weights and free weights. We've come a long way in twenty-five years.) The article quotes one owner saying that when he started lifting weights in college in the 1940s, "Everyone thought it was crazy. Everyone told me it was bad."

Even then, however, in that 1993 article, some still preached against free weights: Phoenix Cardinals strength and conditioning coach Bob Rogucki said athletes lifting free weights were "playing Russian roulette." And, he added, "Some guys are good at it because of their genetic makeup . . . If the exercise excludes the quarterback, then the offensive linemen shouldn't use it."

To be clear, what he was saying there was, basically, that if quarterbacks don't bench-press, then neither should offensive linemen.

Another coach, Washington's Dan Riley, agreed: "The most important aspect for an athlete is his genetics."

Even then, lifting was optional—plenty of NFL players didn't lift, and that was *normal*. George writes, "Nearly everyone agrees that consistency and full participation throughout the year, even in season, offer the best results."

Nearly everyone agrees that consistent weight lifting was important. *Nearly* everyone thinks you should lift some weights *even in season*.

It's like reading about a parallel universe.

Now athletes and their trainers are starting to talk about the brain the way Giants strength and conditioning coach Al Miller did back then. Brandon Payne unknowingly echoed Miller all these years later: "The bottom line has to be this: What am I doing to help the player? . . . What good is it if a team is paying a player five million dollars and his body falls apart?"

Since athletes started lifting weights and taking their cardio seriously, of course, we have seen explosions of greatness within sports, and athletes today look like gods compared to those of fifty years ago. And it's all because sports embraced something once thought strange, confusing—and even dangerous.

Chapter 13

Gaming the Brain

You might not believe it, but as I was delighted to learn, science has found that playing video games can boost performance. Some research about fast-paced first-person shooters like *Halo, Call of Duty,* and the like indicates that they can enhance cognitive function, particularly attention, focus, reaction time, and task switching.

So hey, go get your gamer on.

More delightful still, I have also found a few companies taking advantage of these concepts, engineering games with the explicit purpose of helping athletes—among others—improve their brains, and thus their performance, by building them around the concept of *neuroplasticity*.

NEUROTRACKER

Cristiano Ronaldo, the great striker for Real Madrid and the Portugal national team, moves into the box from a far corner, homing in on the airborne ball that a passer just crossed his way. A beautiful feed to set up the header. The cross reaches its crest and—the lights cut off and everything goes pitch-black. There's a thud. The lights turn back on. The ball rolls into the net.

This is all part of a performance Ronaldo gave as a demonstration about the importance of information processing and cognitive decision making. I watch it in Montreal, on the laptop of Jean Castonguay, CEO of CogniSens, the company whose offices Mindroom's Pierre Beauchamp and I used to turn me into a lab rat. CogniSens sells NeuroTracker, the computer game designed to measure and train cognitive processing.

The three of us now sit in Castonguay's office on a leather couch. Castonguay, a vivacious man with glasses, a stocky, athletic build, and a constant smile, has made everyone espressos and seems to have had a few himself. He points to the screen, excited. "This," he says, "is the epitome of *I got just enough information to put the ball in the net.*"

The video goes to replay, using night vision, to show us how, even after the lights went out, Ronaldo still tracked the ball effortlessly and then executed a beautiful header to send the ball into the net—even though he couldn't possibly have seen it.

NeuroTracker was engineered as a tool for athletes to train up their ability to process more information more quickly. "The idea here," Castonguay says, "is for the more advanced guys to understand that, if you are processing information faster, you're *seizing* information faster, and if you *seize* information faster, you'll be able to *relate* to it faster—which means that a few visual cues will be enough for you to understand what's going on. And if you can capture that *fast,* then you've got an edge on everybody else, because you know more of what's going on."

NeuroTracker, remember, functions like a high-tech shell game on steroids: using a big 3-D TV and 3-D goggles, you track three out of six balls—or four out of eight—which fly around in 3-D for eight seconds at a time. Sessions typically last about ten minutes, and you're scored between about 1.0 and 4.0 depending on how well you do and the level you reach in speed, which an algorithm increases or decreases the better you do.

The game trains up one's information processing and, with variations on the program, decision-making abilities as well.

Castonguay says that the ability to quickly process information and make good decisions is what separated the likes of Wayne Gretzky and Michael Jordan from their peers: "They were smaller than some guys, shorter than some guys, slower than some guys—but they could *see* the game better than anybody else. And, consequently, make better decisions."

He can't tell me *everyone* who's using NeuroTracker, but he shows me a couple of significant examples—the Golden State Warriors, the Oregon University football team during its Chip Kelly–era run of greatness. But that's all Castonguay can say. "We have to be careful when we mention teams and all that," he says. "We've signed so many confidentiality agreements."

The company treats this information with the same hard-core secrecy as the various military folks CogniSens has contracted with, such as Special Forces and Special Ops groups in both the U.S. and Canadian militaries. "[Those] are the worst!" Castonguay says good-naturedly. "Basically they'll make you give them your firstborn if you talk—and they know how to take it!"

Some other folks told me that the San Antonio Spurs and the New England Patriots use NeuroTracker. Matt Ryan, the Atlanta Falcons quarterback, is into it. I've also been told it's being used by Red Bull Racing in England, the Vancouver Canucks, and the Providence College hockey team, which won the 2015 NCAA Championship. Also, IMG Academy, which trains athlete prospects, especially in football, uses it, and the NFL added it to the

Combine's psych evaluation. Some analysts have called for it to replace, or at least somehow merge with, the Wonderlic, the football IQ test.

NeuroTracker was created in 2009 after some members of the Manchester United staff took a ten-hour flight from England to Montreal to visit the Visual Perception and Psychophysics Laboratory at the University of Montreal. Lab director Dr. Jocelyn Faubert has spent two decades researching, among other things, the importance of "sports-related perceptual-cognitive expertise [in] top-level competitive sports," as he said in one of his papers.

In other words, he studies how important it is for athletes to make sense out of what they're seeing.

Manchester's staffers wanted to see if Faubert could build something that their players could use to train in making decisions on the fly, in-game, under high pressure.

Faubert identified four key features: multiple object tracking, large visual field, speed thresholds, and stereoscopic coordination (that is, processing of various depths of vision, such as a basketball being passed your direction while also recognizing the defender coming at you from behind the ball).

With the help of a team of software engineers and others, and after much trial and error, Faubert had a crude version of what the NeuroTracker is today.

The whole idea, as with much of The Stuff in this section, is to overload the brain's cognitive resources, mimicking the same kind of information overload that happens during elite competition. It's the same concept as lifting weights. The more strain, the stronger you grow.

And, also like weight training, you can modify the way you train with NeuroTracker in several ways. The program doesn't stop with the shell game. NeuroTracker training begins with a "consolidation phase"—your brain making sense of this new thing and figuring out what to do with it. Most folks start with six balls and work up to eight.

Athletes rarely sit in chairs while training with NeuroTracker—once they get a handle on the program, they'll use NeuroTracker while standing, and then maybe throw in a balance device, like those half-exercise balls half-balance trays.

And then they'll mix in all other kinds of physical tasks, which CogniSens calls the "dual-task phase." Hockey players train while skating on treadmills, and when they master this, they add in puck handling. Basketball players train while dribbling, football players while doing various footwork drills, baseball players while swinging a bat, shooters while aiming their gun. Some athletes use NeuroTracker in their gyms and lift weights while training.

The only limits, really, are the athletes' and their trainers' resources, space, and imagination.

They can also use a supplementary NeuroTracker program called Optic Flow, with a checkered tunnel pattern behind the floating balls. This makes tracking the correct balls much more difficult, because now you're trying to follow them against a moving, multicolored background instead of a simple black background.

Beyond *that,* there's the "tactical awareness phase": tracking the balls while also analyzing a scene that appears in the background—for example, a quarterback reading defenses, or an Army guy moving through jungle brush with people popping out from behind grass and trees, having to decide whether to shoot if they're an enemy or not shoot if they're on his side or a civilian.

After training with NeuroTracker, athletes frequently report dramatically lower levels of stress come game time. "When you stress," Beauchamp says, "tunnel vision kicks in. That's no good for an athlete. You need to see as much of the field of play as possible."

Reducing stress, on the other hand, turns an athlete's field of vision into what feels like a panorama, because the athlete can take in more information than before.

Faubert wasn't content to just create NeuroTracker and then run with it as a business venture. Sure, he and the university spurred the creation of CogniSens in order to explore Neuro-Tracker's commercial potential—and establish a corporate arm for the university's future research, too—but Faubert is a pure scientist at heart, so he set about studying how NeuroTracker training helped people.

His results were what convinced Castonguay to come on as CEO. Castonguay was a corporate lawyer until 1999, then got involved with a tech start-up, and has been helping grow one tech start-up after another ever since. When UM asked him to help launch CogniSens a few years ago, he said no at first—one of the first technologies he learned they were researching was something that could maybe detect Alzheimer's early, and that felt bleak to Castonguay. "If there's no cure yet," he says, "who wants to know early?"

But he hit it off with Faubert, who started showing him his NeuroTracker research.

In one paper, Faubert reveals a stunning research experiment that compared the cognitive abilities of young twentysomethings and seventysomethings. All active, all healthy, no neurodegenerative diseases to speak of, all that. Faubert split them into a test group and a control group, conducted a proper scientific experiment—control versus experimental, meaning that the control group got something that wasn't the actual thing, while the experimental group got the actual thing. They went through twenty sessions of NeuroTracker training—so twenty sets of twenty rounds, basically, for about fifteen minutes per session. That's it.

Then they looked at how each participant performed in cognitive assessment before training versus after. The seventy-year-olds in the experimental group improved substantially—in fact, they improved to the level of the twenty-year-old control group.

Meanwhile, the twenty-year-old experimental group also improved. Not as dramatically as the seventy-year-old group, but then, when you're twenty years old, your brain and your cognitive abilities are peaking, Faubert and Castonguay reasoned. "So on one hand, they were only slightly better," Castonguay says. "But on the other hand, when it comes to high performance, 'slightly' is huge. That's a competitive advantage, when you're dealing with people that are high-end performers."

As Faubert continued his research, slowly—most things happen slowly in science—he pivoted to studying athletes directly. In 2012, he published a groundbreaking paper in the *Journal of Clinical Sports Psychology,* "Perceptual-Cognitive Training of Athletes," based on research he conducted with two English Premier League soccer teams, three NHL teams, and two rugby teams. He had several dynamic findings. One, the brains of elite athletes are fundamentally different from those of "sub-elite" athletes, even high-level amateurs. He found that elite athletes are already way, way better at filtering out unnecessary information and knowing exactly what to do with the information they take in.

The paper *also* explored whether an athlete could train him or herself to enhance that ability—"increasing perceptual-cognitive thresholds."

And Faubert found that they absolutely could.

He's transparent about the fact that he has to keep most of his data from these elite teams confidential; even so, he saw a clear trend that indicated that most athletes were consistently able to improve. And that surprised him.

Faubert assumed the athletes would *not* improve to a significant degree because they were already the best in the world at what they did. Instead, he saw some hockey players still improve by as much as 40 percent after fifteen sessions. This, he hypothesized, would translate to on-field performance as training with the NeuroTracker expands the athletes' visual fields, meaning they can monitor, say, four players' movements after previously managing only three.

And so all of that is, more or less, what all these supersecretive athletes and teams are using, same as what Manchester United took back to England.

In addition to precompetition training, NeuroTracker provides a means of measuring how ready athletes are come game day. Castonguay says, "If you're not going to be able to perform, the first thing that's going to happen is your cognitive ability's going to drop."

The big 3-D NeuroTracker is their first and primary product, but CogniSens has developed a 2-D iPad app as well. "So while you're traveling, you can train," Beauchamp says.

Beauchamp says some hockey teams use the iPad app to test their goalies before each game in order to get "their neurocognitive score." In other words, which goalie's feeling good? "And if I have a goalie that's off," Beauchamp says, "you know, that's the information the coach is looking for."

Another unexpected benefit for Manchester United was how the NeuroTracker helped their older players. One season after starting to work with NeuroTracker, the club suffered many injuries and ended up with late-thirtysomething players forced to play far more than expected, but who nevertheless managed to keep up. These players later told Castonguay that they felt like NeuroTracker was a big part of their performance, recycling stamina they didn't know they still had.

Yet another surprising benefit of NeuroTracker was how it helped athletes manage injuries better and return from them faster. One Manchester United player got hurt one season and had to sit out several weeks, but during his rehabilitation process, he made sure to spend practice time doing NeuroTracker. When the player came back, after making his brain practice so much complex motion processing, even in an "artificial" way, he was much sharper than most players are after returning from an injury—nowhere near as rusty, and taking much less time to readapt to the speed of the game.

Beauchamp's work with the NeuroTracker had another surprising upside. Remember, athletes often grieve over injuries as one would over losing a loved one. A large reason why has to do with their isolation from the team. (Their identity is often their sport, after all.) In that isolation, they feel less like a teammate.

The injured Manchester player, for instance, made sure to go to the field for his rehab work, and did his NeuroTracker training there while the team was practicing. He saw his teammates, they saw him, they all arrived and left still, more or less, as a unit. "He insisted on it," Castonguay says. "On coming in and doing it when the guys were playing on the field."

"So by staying part of the team," Beauchamp says, "and staying engaged, this guy couldn't be physical for a long time, but by being mentally exercised, he was absolutely capable."

He also became amazingly skilled at the NeuroTracker—his teammates were already capable of scoring an amazing 4.0, but with all of his extra work, he scored a 6.0.

That baffled even Beauchamp. When I asked him how someone can even get a 6.0, Beauchamp smiled and said, "I don't know. It's the subconscious mind being able to do it—if you can trust it."

BRAINHQ

In February 2014, lawyer-turned-businessman Jeff Zimman, a chairman and the former president and CEO at Posit Science, was going through another day at the office in San Francisco when he got a phone call from Patriots quarterback Tom Brady.

Well, technically, he says; it was actually Tom Brady's personal trainer, Alex Guerrero. But Guerrero was calling to say Brady wanted a meeting.

Zimman laughs about it now. He says, "Alex basically explained who he was and that he had a team of neuroscientists, and they were using our exercises, and Tom wanted to talk to somebody here."

And what Brady most wanted to talk about was BrainHQ, Posit Science's computer-based brain-training system comprising twenty-nine different video games engineered in accordance with scientific research in order to enhance everything from working memory to peripheral vision, all by playing video games on a computer.

A few days after Guerrero's phone call, Zimman and a few other members of the Posit Science team flew out to Boston. "We were kind of blown away by what they had been up to up there," Zimman says.

When I ask him to elaborate, he laughs and says, "I will leave that as a story for them to tell."

As it turns out, Brady and his team decline to tell that story. When I e-mail the Patriots' media relations guy to try setting something up, he says, "Tom's going to do what he does best— PASS!"

I even go to Foxboro myself to visit the TB12 training center Brady has built beside the Patriots' stadium. They also decline.

(This is not unlike many such attempts I made over the course of my little quest, with many other athletes for many other products.)

But of course, as with all athletes using any of This Stuff, Brady thinks it's this brand-new cutting-edge competitive edge, when, as it turns out, it's been around for a good while now.

Elite athletes weren't even on the radar for Zimman and Posit Science before the Brady meetings. At least not elite athletes in mainstream sports; military outfits had been using Posit Science and BrainHQ products for years in order to shore up their soldiers' cognitive abilities.

BrainHQ's exercises were originally designed to help children with ADHD and other learning disabilities, and to help an aging population keep their brains sharp and stave off typical struggles with driving, memory, and so on.

Controversy has shadowed Posit Science and BrainHQ, which many compare to Lumosity, the "brain-training" company that lied to people by telling them playing their brain-training video games could prevent Alzheimer's and such. Lumosity got hit with a $50 million fine by the FTC in January 2016. (That amount was later reduced to $2 million.)

However, BrainHQ has two big factors to consider that made me stop and reconsider.

First, their founder, Dr. Michael Merzenich. You might remember him. He's the relentless neuroscientist who proved neuroplasticity and revealed to all of us that we can change. He had other ideas once he changed the world, and one was to start BrainHQ.

Zimman himself—who sounds every bit like a classic good company pitchman on the phone—says that when Merzenich came to him with the BrainHQ concept decades ago, he was as skeptical as anyone criticizing them now. Zimman was a lawyer, and before that, a philosophy major, then a newspaper reporter, and then became so obsessed with tech that he went to law *and* business school at Stanford. When he finished those, he joined a small San Francisco law firm, and figured he'd practice law a couple years, then work on launching and building companies. Fourteen years later, he'd become a partner, helped the firm grow from sixty attorneys to more than eight hundred, and he was running its San Francisco office. He thought he'd be there for life.

Then, one Friday afternoon in 1995, he had his meeting with Merzenich, who came in with an MBA student from Berkeley. Merzenich wanted Zimman's advice about a company, Scientific Learning, he wanted to start that made video games that kids could play to get smarter. "I have to admit, I was kind of looking at my watch," Zimman says. He hadn't realized that Merzenich was a neuroscience rock star, and Zimman heard pie-in-the-sky, pseudoscientific delusions every day, and this sounded like another one. He was coasting, waiting for their hour to end, when Merzenich said, "Is there any reason to incorporate the company before our article appears in *Science*?"

Science is a highly respected magazine published by the nonprofit American Association for the Advancement of Science. Zimman didn't know *much* about them, but he knew getting something published in the magazine was a big deal. "And actually," Merzenich said, "it's the cover story. It'll appear in about three or four weeks."

Zimman said they needed to start talking to venture capitalists pronto.

All of BrainHQ's concepts are based on the concept of neuroplasticity, and Merzenich's goal with Scientific Learning was to present a new way of teaching, taking his research on the plasticity of the brain and applying it to concepts that could help children learn. His mother's first cousin was an elementary school teacher in Wisconsin and she once won teacher of the year for the whole United States. Merzenich's mother, he recalls, asked her what her most important principles were for successful teaching. His cousin said, "You test them when they come into school, and you figure out whether they are worthwhile. And if they are worthwhile, you really pay attention to them, and you don't waste time on the ones that aren't."

That answer shocked Merzenich. He later said, "And that's reflected in how people have treated children who are different forever. It's just so destructive."

Merzenich knew that children—all children—could always become more intelligent. His research, remember, had proven that anyone's brain could be changed, and if it could be changed, it could be improved.

All of this led him to Zimman's law offices that day.

He told Zimman that he wanted to use his knowledge to solve some sort of human problem, or even several, and wanted to start with children. Language-learning deficits, dyslexia, ADD and ADHD, that sort of stuff. He developed video games designed (1) to be fun, and (2), most importantly, to address the underlying issues such children faced.

The company launched in 1996, went public in 1999, and has since helped some seven million kids, its games apparently having significant impact on their ability to better focus in school.

Along the way, however, Merzenich wanted to help *more* than children. If the brain could be changed at any age, there had to be more they could do for way more people.

So, in 2003, he went back to Zimman, who'd since left the law firm for an investment bank that threw a bunch of money at him, then left *that* for a sabbatical, then quit the sabbatical to take a part-time job at a venture firm. Merzenich asked him to dinner, during which he raved about what his research showed, and how well Scientific Learning was doing, and how much more he wanted to do. "And for a scientist," Zimman says, "Mike's a really good sales guy, because he closed with, 'It would be criminal if you didn't come help me do this.'"

After a couple weeks of due-diligence research, Zimman decided to join up with Merzenich. They started Posit Science in 2003, in Zimman's basement. Even though it was, in Zimman's words, "the nuclear winter of venture capital," they managed to raise $7 million to start the company. And along the way, Zimman says, Merzenich "was very strategic" in terms of what he told him. "He waited until he had me signed up and working on the business plan before we had our second dinner, and he explained to me that age is really just the tip of the iceberg. He rattled off one neurological condition after another that we should address, and told me about work being done by his students, and his students' students, and their students, and their students, all over the world, that kind of said, we could build exercises that would address a whole host of ills." Zimman laughs. "And I found it all very confusing."

In short, BrainHQ's methods aim to address everything from aging to mental illness to neurodegenerative diseases like Alzheimer's and Parkinson's. Zimman says, "We've been able to show that we could take a normal, healthy aging person and pretty dramatically improve their cognitive abilities."

And here's the second reason I reconsidered BrainHQ: independent studies have shown that their stuff works.

One such study of about five hundred people conducted by the Mayo Clinic found that BrainHQ's various video-game exercises improved information processing, attention, and memory by a quarter of a standard deviation—or about ten years. In other words, proper training with BrainHQ video games appeared to turn back the clock on people's brains by about a decade.

One game, Double Decision, involves splitting the screen and then identifying which vehicle is on the road while also locating a

Route 66 sign wherever it appears. This tremendously helped seniors with their driving by increasing their "useful field of view." Basically this means you can quickly—and accurately—see details when looking straight ahead. The larger, the better. This is an ability that tends to shrink with age, but BrainHQ exercises like Double Decision help enhance it.

There have been more than one hundred research papers independently written and reviewed by the scientific community and then published in scientific journals that seem to pretty solidly point to the soundness of BrainHQ's products and their claims. That is, after all, what got Tom Brady's attention.

They'd heard people say BrainHQ helped improve their bowling scores and tennis games and such, but Brady was the first "real" athlete they'd heard of using BrainHQ, let alone expressing so much interest. Zimman says, "We had never focused on the fact that you know, in most sports, that milliseconds, fractions of seconds, and inches, actually matter. Especially on an elite level. That's the difference between the person who wins and the person who loses. And we're all about improving performance by tenths and thousandths of seconds."

After Brady's phone call back in February 2014, Zimman says, "Basically we realized that these same things would improve anybody's skills."

Now Zimman regularly has meetings with elite athletic organizations, same as the meetings he's had with countless other companies. BrainHQ *does* sell to consumers, sure, and if you visit their websites, they look like a straight-to-consumer company, but the other half of their business is business-to-business. Zimman says they work a lot with auto insurance companies such as State Farm, USAA, AAA, and more, as well as health insurance companies and long-term-care insurance companies.

The difference between what a sports team needs to know and

what those insurance companies want is hilarious. To meet with an insurance company, Zimman has to block out the entire afternoon. Sports teams? Only fifteen minutes, and if they're interested, maybe about fifteen minutes of demo, tops. Typically his intro is a six-to-ten-slide PowerPoint presentation, but most teams only have time for one slide, so he usually goes with one headlined "BrainHQ and Enhanced Performance."

The slide highlights a dozen different items—processing speed, reaction time, visual acuity, visual search, multiple object tracking, useful field of view, peripheral vision, attention, memory, executive function, balance, and mobility—and includes a few graphics, one of which indicates that BrainHQ training can double the players' visual speed of processing. The slide says, "The exercises take a baseline for each athlete and track and report on improvements across hours of training. These measurements include the split-second improvements in speed and reaction time that translate into success on the field, as well as percentile gains in attention, memory, intelligence, and other cognitive functions."

The slide displays three more graphics showing how BrainHQ can cut athletes' reaction times in half, make them 25 percent better at tracking multiple objects, and expand their field of vision by 200 percent.

"And," Zimman says, "they get it. *It's gonna make my brain split seconds faster, and it's gonna make it inches more accurate.* And when I'm talking to people in Europe at FIFA, I get to say 'millimeters' and 'milliseconds,' which I really like."

After athletes try BrainHQ for a while, Zimman will ask for feedback, and he says the most common response is that they feel like they can see things more quickly and react faster, and this means that the game slows down for them, too.

The one hundred scientific papers and all the seemingly quantified results BrainHQ has produced are impressive, but none of these have had anything to do directly with sports. That's the only issue that leaves me feeling leery. Not that my opinion matters all that much when Tom Brady is so ardently bought in, but still, BrainHQ's products frequently feel like little more than playing video games. No matter how scientifically engineered someone claims something is, as a former athlete, I find it difficult to wrap my mind around the idea that a video game that has nothing to do with football can help someone be better at football.

I am far from the first person to think this. That perception is one of the predominant problems faced by companies like BrainHQ. It is difficult to convince people about the concept of "transferability." Some of those one hundred papers, after all, claim that BrainHQ's cognitive skills are indeed transferable to, say, a seventy-five-year-old when she gets into her own car. But they don't say this about playing quarterback.

I e-mail Greg Appelbaum, the Duke neuroscientist, again, and ask him what he thinks.

He tells me he's been using BrainHQ exercises in some of his classes and research, but even then, he replies, "I'm still skeptical. BrainHQ has more science traction than Lumosity, but they are effectively doing the same things. There are subtle differences, but if [programs like them] work, they all work. If one is garbage, they are all garbage. Of course, Lumosity got slammed by the FTC and the others haven't, but that is because of marketing more than the games or the science. As for the science, it is an open question if these tools work or if they are better than other uses of time (learning a new language, exercise, etc.)."

I tell him about Tom Brady and the other athletes who seem to love BrainHQ and feel like they're getting results: Could that be legit? Appelbaum will only say, "I wouldn't be surprised if some guy tells you that. And I wouldn't be surprised if Tom Brady thinks it works."

Chapter 14

Training Times One Hundred

Where video-game training like NeuroTracker, BrainHQ, and the like strengthens the mind by strengthening the brain's cognitive processing in a way that—ideally—translates to the field, others have taken the concepts in those games and applied them directly to sports video games themselves. That is, they have created video games that enable athletes to train within the sport itself, like Madden on steroids.

AXON SPORTS

EXOS is a gigantic gym and state-of-the-art training facility in Phoenix, Arizona, and the flagship location for the greater EXOS brand. It is also one of the premier destinations for elite athletes and aspiring elite athletes. There are millions of dollars' and fifty tons' worth of fitness equipment to keep the body strong. Dozens of athletes lift, grunt, yell, cringe, hurt, sweat, and sweat some more, not an ounce more fat than necessary on the lot of them.

Hard to believe that a few decades ago, this wasn't even expected of athletes.

On the second floor, there is a modest room with a large window overlooking the floor below. The decor in this room is striking. On the wall, there is a fifty-five-inch touch-screen monitor, on which athletes play video games that have been engineered by Axon Sports. Their motto: "Train Above the Neck."

Football players can put themselves into just about any scheme imaginable. Want to get some reps in at quarterback, get a feel for how a defense shifts to cover a blitz? You got it. Want to be in that defense, maybe outside linebacker? Or safety? There you go. There are presnap and just-postsnap simulations—against players that look like actual human beings, which they are, not video-game characters—for virtually every position. Quarterback, running back, tight end, offensive lineman. Defensive lineman. Linebacker. Cornerback. As position specific as you could want.

Baseball players can essentially see live pitching from just about any professional pitcher.

After logging in and selecting which pitcher they want to face—there are more than a dozen options—they stand in front of the monitor in a batting stance. The pitcher on the screen looks almost exactly like he'd look if they were standing on an actual baseball field. The background looks like a real stadium. There are tall pitchers, short pitchers, right-handers, left-handers, overhand throwers, sidearm throwers, and just about everything in between. They throw 100 mph. They throw wicked breaking balls. They throw everything that a hitter in the majors would see.

And it's all customizable, as random or as controlled as you want.

The batter doesn't swing like in batting practice; the goal here isn't contact, but pitch recognition. When the pitches come in, the batter reaches out and presses a button on the screen to identify what type of pitch he just saw. He's scored on how accurate he is as well as how quickly he responds. The better he does, the more difficult the game gets.

When the pitcher winds and fires, he looks like a real person, not an awkward video-game version of a person, because he is a real person. He's an athlete-slash-actor who has been filmed by Axon.

One of Axon's core goals is the same as much of The Stuff in this section: use scientifically engineered technology to slow the game down for athletes, helping them become more quick, efficient, and accurate at making high-speed decisions.

Axon's only been around about six years, and its products are still rare but increasingly in demand; a few consumer models are available but most are secreted away in the facilities of elite sports organizations around the world. The company primarily focuses on baseball and American football right now, though they also work in softball, cricket, rugby, and soccer.

I visit company president Jason Sada at Axon headquarters in early 2016. Theirs is a modest setup in the middle of a large Scottsdale office complex, about twenty minutes from EXOS. Sada greets me at the door holding a big cup of coffee and smiling. Friendly and highly caffeinated. He flew back to town last night, and he's back on a plane tomorrow.

There's a bookshelf front and center, a few baseball and football helmets sitting on top, painted matte black with Axon logos on the side. Beneath them: three huge binders labeled *BRAIN RESEARCH,* filled with more than a thousand pages' worth of papers, diagrams, graphs, and more. The science concerning the Axon products themselves is still developing, but they are engineered around what science says works best. The binders have subtitles like *Emotional Regulation; Focus & Imagination; Concussion, General; Executive Function & Split Attention; People of Interest; Spatial Reasoning & Chunking; Visual Cues & Anticipation; High-Speed Decision Making;* and *Myelin.*

Sada himself is no scientist—he has scientists working for him—but a businessman. He worked at Intel for a long time, then started a couple other companies before getting introduced to what eventually became Axon. As we talk, I learn that he's obsessed with making Axon work because before he was a businessman, he, too, was an athlete. He played club soccer at New Mexico State, and playing soccer made him ask questions.

There had to be ways to get better. The primary way that athletes had worked on improving their game was by brute force. Go to the field, the batting cage, the arena, wherever, and physically practice what you want to practice until you've done enough reps to feel improved, coach or trainer guiding you along, all that. He wondered if it was possible to do the repetitions you needed to do without putting that kind of strain on your actual body.

He also wondered if there was a viable alternative to film, both for working on one's own game and for studying opponents. Players and coaches, especially at the elite levels, spend hours studying film; those in football notoriously spend nearly full workweeks' worth of time watching their opponents.

I videoed myself hitting and throwing starting in eighth grade and juxtaposed it, over and over, with films of the guys I wanted to play like. Mike Piazza was a favorite hitter, Iván Rodríguez a favorite catcher. And my mom videotaped every single one of my games, so I would study pitchers before I faced them again, too.

The obvious limitation of this approach, though, is exactly what Sada says he was thinking back when he was in college: "Watching film was such a passive activity."

Sada wanted to combine the benefits of visualization with

those of watching film. "When you rehearsed these things mentally, they felt familiar in a game situation," he says. "Again, as an
eighteen-year-old, I didn't know anything, but I always felt that
sports and technology need to come up with ways to help athletes
get more of that experience—more ways to engage in the learning
process outside of the field."

Axon's products are too new to have received the thorough
scrutiny required to validate their efficacy, something that can
take years and years. In terms of the science world, Axon has just
been born. But the worth of their products is measured in terms
of helping teams, and clearly, teams and athletes are starting to
buy in.

It took some convincing for Sada to tell me who he's working
with even *off* the record. I'll say this, though—the names of the
teams he did reveal, off the record, are some of the best in the
world. The Axon staff flies in and goes directly to these teams'
facilities and spends weeks setting up the Axon gear and then cus-
tomizing the software in excruciatingly minute detail so that, by
the time they're done, the whole setup looks like something the
team created and branded themselves. It's their logo on everything, their colors, their defensive schemes and pitching information and so on—the process sounds almost overly thought out,
incredibly rigorous, expensive, and time-consuming.

Any athlete worth anything could use one such product and
know immediately if it will help them or not, and it seems like a
lot of teams and players are using Axon quite a bit. During my
visit, Sada told me that as of then—early 2016—they had about
2.5 million recorded practice reps in the Axon system across all
their sports. A great deal of those are coming from the pros using
their program.

"We see players who are new to a team quickly producing,"
Sada says. "And saying, 'It's helping me learn how to play in this

scheme, how to play in this system.' We've also . . . run comparisons of performance in games when they've done higher volumes of training versus when they do less. And we see that the results are different. I firmly believe in the athletes' self-assessment. And in particular, when an athlete comes into a team that they haven't played with but they are a great athlete, in my opinion, the biggest hurdle is a cognitive one. Like, if this person has all the tools to be a great fill-in-the-blank player, but has never played for Team A, let's quickly leverage all that experience and everything they've developed up to this point to also replicate it with exactly what you want them to do with Team A. And then we hear those people are always our earliest adopters. They get into it. Because it's a tool that's helping them become a producer for that team."

The EXOS unit was the first one out in the wild a few years ago; Axon started its public life collecting data from some of the best football prospects going through EXOS—then called Athletes' Performance—including the likes of now–NFL quarterbacks Andrew Luck and Robert Griffin III.

In 2014, one of Axon's clients, the University of Oregon, *did* give some interviews to *USA Today,* and they raved about it. They were Axon's first college football team, starting when Chip Kelly was still their head coach. Current head coach Mark Helfrich told the paper that some players used Axon more than others, depending on position, but a good number used it every day.

Marcus Mariota, the Oregon quarterback who went on to win the Heisman and is now a rising star in the NFL, told the paper that Axon helped him with protections, identifying zone blitzes, and made him sharper at finding linebackers. He said, "It's a great tool . . . that really provides you a lot of good tools that you can use to help yourself."

Oregon offensive coordinator Scott Frost agreed, saying that Axon had helped Mariota and the team on the whole, saying the best part was simply "putting that kind of pressure on guys off the field as well as on the field."

One of Sada's favorite success stories is a minor league baseball team we'll just call the Bashers. (As with all companies, Sada can't talk publicly about most of the teams he works with.) The first season the Bashers used Axon, the number of home runs they hit nearly tripled. (And even that information is something I had to pry out of Sada.) He says, "Of course, can we say on every team they're going to get two hundred percent improvements in home runs? No, certainly not. We're never going to come out and claim that, because that was just literally probably one or two people who needed that skill to be developed, and are great hitters. These weren't slackers who never hit a ball. And so it's just that misperception that we want to avoid . . . But our baseball numbers, they're absurdly high. The end-game results in better contact for everybody."

Axon's allure to athletes and teams is more understandable to me than maybe anything else in this section. No, Axon probably wouldn't have helped me throw the ball back to the pitcher or make better defensive decisions, but I can easily see how Axon would have given me more confidence at the plate, which I can then see transferring into the rest of my game, which maybe helps me relax more on the field. Who knows? But anything that makes you more confident is going to make you a better player. After all, to quote Yogi Berra, "Ninety percent of the game is half mental."

Axon might not have the scientific studies of, say, BrainHQ to back it up, but they're also totally different in scope. What Axon boils down to is simple: they've designed a gorgeous software program that gives athletes more reps, and seriously cut into that 10,000-Hour (or Whatever) Rule problem of physical wear and tear. One of Axon's key employees, former NFL quarterback Joe

Germaine, says getting just a hundred reps on the field would take two days' worth of practice. Using Axon, quarterbacks can get a hundred and fifty solid reps in ten minutes.

Sada says that a lot of the pro teams and elite college teams he's working with have said this is a real problem. "In the NFL and college football . . . where they're not going full speed and making contact—the challenge is, they are going to go full speed on Saturday and Sunday," Sada says. "So your brain hasn't seen high-speed decisions and hasn't seen full speed, then all of a sudden it does [see them] in the most critical environment where everyone's going full speed . . . ? And there's risk of other injuries."

In an era where the awareness of traumatic brain injury and concussion is growing all the time, the type of training Axon promises is even more important. You get the mental gain that comes from repetition without the physical risk.

Practice isn't exactly endangered by Axon either, but then, Axon's goal isn't to replace practice in the first place, any more than a strength and conditioning coach would want to replace practice with more weight lifting. "We always joke that recognizing pitches *is* an incredible tool—if you can hit a baseball," Sada says. "I mean the reality is, if you want to be a baseball player, you have to be able to hit a ball. And you better have great bat speed, and you better have hand-eye coordination. You better have all these tools in your box. But in addition to that, you should be able to recognize the pitch type. None of this is in a vacuum. Now we always talk about 'train above the neck' because we isolate that part."

On top of all of this, Axon's work seems held in high regard by the biggest name in sports: Nike. The company worked with Axon to integrate some of their ideas, with the help of developer AKQA in London, to develop Nike Pro Genius, a slick new brain-training app the explicit goal of which is, according to Nike's release, "to destigmatize and democratize mental training."

The app—located within the Nike Soccer app—feels half Axon, half psychologist. Highlighting a dozen or so elite soccer players, some of whom even narrate parts of the app, Nike Pro Genius walks players through an array of mental training, including decision making, strategy, confidence, and more. It uses five primary tools and techniques: priming, counterattack, crossing—athletic tasks that take users through an array of various in-game situations—and the psychological tools of visualization and self-talk.

The ad for it had the usual Nike feel, all athletic and cool and inspirational, featuring some of the sports world's biggest soccer stars, including Cristiano Ronaldo, but there was a wrinkle to it: these athletes didn't appear to actually be *doing* anything—they were staring into their smartphones and there were vivid neon lines and sparks flashing in overlays of their head and down their spines and through their limbs. "What separates the good from the truly great?" asks a British, super-epic voice-over. "The world's best train their brain like a muscle. They are geniuses."

NEUROSCOUTING

In a New York City office, I'm using an iPhone that Jason Sherwin just handed me to play a pitch-identification baseball game sort of like Axon's. Sherwin is the scruffy thirtysomething founder and CEO of deCervo, a start-up in the budding field of "neuroscouting." It's exactly what it sounds like. Some teams are taking Axon-like concepts, devising their own proprietary programs, and marketing them as, among other things, a way to evaluate prospects.

Maybe the most famous neuroscouting story right now is that of Mookie Betts, the Boston Red Sox outfielder who has been taking the league by storm. As I write this, he's just hit his fifth home run in two games to become just one of three Red Sox players to ever do that, including Nomar Garciaparra and Carl Yastrzemski. And Mookie's a *little* guy, a trim five-foot-nine.

In 2011, he started participating in a neuroscouting evaluation program the Red Sox were trying to implement. Theirs came from a company called, well, NeuroScouting, based in nearby Cambridge. This was supposed to be a secret, but the *Boston Globe* dug it up.

I met with the NeuroScouting guys, Brian Miller and Wes Clapp, in Cambridge the day after my meeting with Sherwin in New York. Miller and Clapp met by pure coincidence in San Francisco in 2006, when they were both doing postdoc work, and had the idea to start a company using brain-training science and tech to improve player performance. Though their name is, you know, NeuroScouting, and they do scouting work now, they started as a performance-enhancing company, and they also work in the health care sector, having scored some grants from the National Institutes of Health to study various neurological conditions.

They're great to talk with about all This Stuff, but they're supersecretive about *their* Stuff. They couldn't even tell me, on the record, how many teams they work with, or what, exactly, they do with them. Clapp says, "Our clients are really wanting us to be this secret edge."

All Miller and Clapp tell me is that they use some EEG to test the validity of their software, which measures things like reaction times and accuracy—sounding pretty similar to deCervo's products—and that they use a "brain computer interface," though they can't give me more details than that. One of the main reasons for this is that, as Miller says, "We share a lot of joint IP with our clients."

They're dipping their toes into basketball and football, but NeuroScouting's main focus has been baseball, specifically hitters. "You see how baseball's evolved," Miller says. "Pitching has gotten so much better, and you have these power arms just dominating, and it's pushing us even further, because basically now they're cutting down the window for the batter. It's always been this battle between a hitter and a pitcher. The pitcher is earning more milliseconds by being more deceptive, becoming faster, and really crunching those decision-making windows. And what we're doing is trying to, for the hitter, get that time back."

The way reporter Alex Speier describes the NeuroScouting program in his February 2015 feature story for the *Boston Globe*, Betts and other prospects, using a laptop, watched pitches on a baseball simulation program, and identified them as fast as they could by tapping a space bar; their score was based on speed and accuracy.

Red Sox scouts drooled over Betts's athleticism—he could dunk a basketball, and in high school, he had played shortstop, second base, and center field with the greatest of ease. He didn't have much power, but he smoked one line drive after another. Beyond that, however, they started to love something else about him, something they called "the workings of his mind." Asked what he meant by that, then–Red Sox general manager Theo Epstein laughed and said, "I can't talk about that stuff because then I'd have to kill you."

Betts got obsessed with the program, even though he thought it was superhard. He would miss lunch to "do neuroscouting." Hard as he thought it was, Betts was among the best at the program in the 2011 draft class. Nobody knew what that meant, exactly, but it compelled the Red Sox to draft him in the fifth round that year. One member of Boston's front office told Speier, "If this guy turns out to be a prospect, we'll know this [expletive] works."

According to that logic, this [expletive] works.

Betts rose fast through the ranks, making his MLB debut within three years of getting drafted. He was twenty-one. "A microwaved career," according to Tom Verducci's 2015 *Sports*

Illustrated profile of the kid. Now twenty-four, Betts mostly plays outfield, and he's become one of Boston's best hitters. What NeuroScouting showed was that Betts has a remarkable ability to recognize pitches quickly, and his brain processes visual information exceptionally well. "He's able to react and see things a little better than the rest," then Red Sox bench coach Torey Lovullo, now the Arizona Diamondbacks' manager, told Speier. "In his pre-draft meetings, he was top of the class [in neuroscouting]. He rated as high as anyone has ever rated."

This concept of neuroscouting has the potential to completely change the way athletes are evaluated. For baseball scouts and coaches, knowing whether a guy can identify a pitch within five feet or twenty-five feet of leaving the pitcher's hand can predict the future.

Lots of stud ballplayers graduate high school rarely if ever having faced pitching faster than 90 mph. In the pros, 90-plus is common.

"Let's say you've got Player A and Player B," says Sherwin. "They both hit .800 in high school, astronomical batting averages. Player A is picking up his pitches about five feet out of the release of the pitcher. Player B, on the other hand, is picking up the pitches at twenty feet or thirty feet. In high school, that difference isn't going to be that big of a deal. Once you start ramping up the speed, ramping up the sharpness of the breaks, when you get to the Major League level, that difference of twenty-five feet in terms of when Player A is making his decision and when Player B is making his decision, that's a big difference."

The Red Sox in 2010 began requiring minor leaguers from class Double A on down to participate in the NeuroScouting program, which takes about fifteen to twenty minutes per session. To keep it fun, they also shared a leaderboard so players could see how they stacked up against their teammates.

As a fun and useful next layer, deCervo also frequently combines the pitch identification software with EEG equipment in order to track exactly *when* the ballplayer's brain makes its decision whether to swing.

Whatever develops with neuroscouting, the timing of companies such as Axon couldn't be better. Putting players on the field in their minds and giving them a comparable experience to actual play without subjecting them to any of the physical tolls and risks? Are you kidding me? Who knows what's going to happen with Axon or any of the rest of these—but they may well be the future of sports.

The NCAA is looking to implement new rules to cut down on physical contact in practice. The Ivy League announced in March 2016 that they were banning tackling in football practice. Concussion and other head-injury concerns are swelling in the NFL. Most severe injuries don't happen on one terrible play, but rather develop because of repeated stress and strain. Many concussions come not from one awful hit, but from many repeated blows to the head. So as high-speed, stressful practice time is reduced, the need for something like what Axon offers is only going to grow.

Ditto for other sports. Games like baseball and basketball and cricket might not have the same physical dangers as football, but they still demand a certain physical grind. It is realistic to speculate that implementing the Axon system could drastically reduce the amount of time athletes have to spend on their feet and in the gym while increasing the amount of reps they get.

The only thing better than playing video games that simulate live game experiences would be if, instead of simply looking *at* a screen of a virtual situation, we could step *into* the screen.

Well, funny I should mention that . . .

Chapter 15

"And Shoot, It's *Real!*"

Heading into June 2015, the Dallas Cowboys hadn't won a Super Bowl in some twenty years, and so they set out to change that by becoming the first team in the NFL to sign a contract with STRIVR Labs, a virtual-reality sports start-up and one of what seem to be at least three different types of virtual reality relevant to my little quest here: headsets, simulators, and caves.

More upscale versions of virtual-reality training have been in use by pilots, surgeons, and other professionals for decades, and there's a wealth of empirical data on how good it is for helping our brains learn and adapt and grow. A Navy study once found that student pilots who used a flight simulator were more likely to score above average in real flight tests compared to their peers who trained without the simulator.

And these flight simulators are *intense.* (Commercial pilots often train on similar simulators.) The simulator sits on top of a hydraulic lift system linked up with the software and reacts according to whatever the pilot is doing, creating roughly the same sensation of tilt and rotation and all that a pilot would experience in the air. This is *haptic feedback*. In a milder form, think of the "rumble packs" you used for old Nintendo 64 and Dreamcast controllers, and the way that pretty much every video-game controller vibrates when you play now. (That word *haptic* comes from the Greek *haptikos*, which means "pertaining to the sense of touch.")

Red Bull last year installed a new Formula 1 racing simulator in its Santa Monica High Performance Center. You sit down, strap in, and are surrounded by three enormous screens that display a hyperrealistic track. The controls in front of you are almost identical to what you'd find in the cockpit of an actual F1 race car. Powerful speakers rev the engine so loud that, even in the lobby on the far opposite side of the massive building, you can still hear it. When you get up to speed, you *feel* it, as the seat rumbles and the engine roars, and you devour the road. And when—not if—you wipe out, Andy Walshe recommends releasing the wheel because the strain of holding on to it can hurt your wrists and shoulders.

And all of that is a *pared-back* version of their full-blown simulator at Red Bull Racing.

Another VR study had eight residents in surgery at a hospital perform an operation in virtual-reality training, and afterward, that group finished a gallbladder dissection 29 percent faster than eight students who didn't train with VR. Other studies have found that VR-based "3-D classrooms" improved 86 percent of students' test scores, and doubled their attention levels, from 50 to 94 percent.

All of that is giving rise to . . . this.

HEADSETS

Carson Palmer is an old man at heart. At thirty-six, he's not exactly a young man in body for the NFL, and fittingly enough, the Cardinals quarterback is notorious among teammates and coaches for his grumpy-old-guy attitude toward all things analog. He takes notes in team meetings with pen and paper, and waves off iPads for old-school stuffed three-ring binders as playbooks.

But around the same time the Cowboys started using STRIVR, Palmer got his hands on one of the headsets, and became the first NFL quarterback to install a STRIVR system in his home. During the 2015–2016 season, he used STRIVR every morning and afternoon, six days a week. In early 2016, he told ESPN that he spent almost as much time on the STRIVR as he did on the team playbook.

STRIVR is an Oculus VR headset that creates 360-degree interactive videos of teams' practices. To do this, at the beginning of the Cardinals' season, the STRIVR team spent a few weeks at training camp, sticking stationary cameras behind the line of scrimmage and elsewhere on the field, then stitched the video together to create the VR version, wherein the quarterback can see anywhere he wants on the field, complete with sound.

Palmer had his best season ever that year. He had career highs in passing yards (4,671, fourth in the league), touchdowns (thirty-five, tied for second in the league), and quarterback rating (104.6, third in the league)—and he led five game-winning drives, the most in the league.

Palmer's backups loved STRIVR, too—typically, second-stringer Drew Stanton got extra "reps" in during practice by standing twenty feet behind Palmer. He'd watch film, too, of both practices and games, but as great a tool as film has been for teams through the years, it's still just film. Using the STRIVR, Stanton essentially stepped into Palmer's cleats as he went through practice. "At eye level," Stanton has raved. "And seeing everything around you. It's such an impressive tool."

Arizona's third-string quarterback, Matt Barkley, joined the team right at the start of the season after a trade, meaning he had zero time to learn a whole new playbook and offensive system. He said STRIVR helped him learn the schemes much faster. "Virtual reps," he called it.

Linebacker Kevin Minter also got obsessed with the STRIVR, using it every day after practice and often coming in early to get extra time. "It changes the whole thing," he's said. And, he added, "It helped me slow it down."

By now, there are six more teams in the NFL using STRIVR's tech, including the Saints, 49ers, Vikings, and Jets. As for the Dallas Cowboys, they dedicated an entire room at their training facility to VR, where it was used primarily by quarterbacks, as well as linebackers and safeties. In the room, the players wore the STRIVR headset connected to a television monitor, so spectators could see what the STRIVR user saw. This way, coaches could tell players to pause, pointing out what they need to see.

Of all the technologically and scientifically difficult things STRIVR does, its greatest challenge may be earning the trust of NFL teams. Think about it—they are creating immersive videos of teams' every play in practice, meaning they become completely familiar with a team's playbook and strategies and all of its most confidential material.

That means convincing not just players to buy in, or even their coaches and trainers, but the entire staff. No easy feat.

That was one of the big hesitations for coaches when STRIVR started bringing their services to them. NFL reporter Bruce Feldman at FoxSports.com wrote a column in March 2015 detailing the almost absurdly secretive way STRIVR was introduced to NFL brass:

During NFL Combine week, downtown Indianapolis swells with little clandestine meetings, where seemingly innocuous details are discussed like matters of national security. There's back-of-the-restaurant gatherings, coffee-shop meet-ups, sit-downs in obscure bars. And, for three consecutive days in late February, there was room 1040 of the Westin hotel.

Coaches from 10 NFL teams—and the GM from an 11th in Denver Broncos legend John Elway—visited room 1040. What they experienced inside the suite, they would later say, was unlike anything they'd ever seen. Their hosts were three men, each around 30 years old: an ex–NFL quarterback; a kicker-turned-MBA/college coach; and a former FBI agent who specialized in counter-terrorism. In the middle of the room were two laptops set together so their screens operated as one. On it was, perhaps, the future of football coaching.

One of the coaches later told Feldman, "I was expecting something kinda cheesy, like video-game quality, and right when I was about to write them off, they put the headset on you, and, shoot, it's *real*."

What then twenty-nine-year-old STRIVR cofounder and CEO Derek Belch showed those coaches was video of a practice at Stanford University. Belch graduated from Stanford in 2008 after attending four years as a kicker for the football team. The way his story goes, in 2007, he took a class with Professor Jeremy Bailenson, founder and director of Stanford's Virtual Human Interaction Lab. He had the idea to create a virtual-reality system that could help athletes better and more quickly prepare for games. Bailenson loved the idea but said that technology hadn't advanced far enough yet to make it real.

Six years later, Belch was a graduate assistant for the Stanford football team and talked with Bailenson again about his idea.

Bailenson told him the technology could handle it now, so it became the focus of Belch's master's thesis. With Bailenson's help, Belch spent two years designing what would become STRIVR's 360-degree immersive video program. His project culminated in Stanford's football team using his program to prepare, over the course of three weeks, for their final three games.

The result: their best three games of the season, capped off by a 45–21 win against Maryland in the Foster Farms Bowl. Stanford coach David Shaw said that what Belch had made was "game-changing."

Belch originally wanted to be a coach, but Shaw urged him to pursue his virtual-reality training concept by starting a company. "If I were you," Shaw told him, "I'd put everything I had into this."

Belch named his company STRIVR for "Sports Training in Virtual Reality," and incorporated in January 2015.

Now the STRIVR team comprises more than a dozen people, including Bailenson and former NFL QB Trent Edwards, both of whom helped cofound it. In addition to the NFL teams, STRIVR has also caught on with twelve college football teams, plus a college basketball team, an NBA team, a WNBA team, and an NHL team.

Maybe I couldn't see what they did for the Cowboys, but Belch pointed me toward a project they undertook in partnership with Google, Bank of America, and Visa to create a fan experience that he said should give me a good idea of what the NFL teams get.

In late 2015, as a way to promote STRIVR and help Google promote its VR products, they filmed with the New England Patriots, and that December, Google gave out ten thousand Google Cardboard VR headsets at Gillette Stadium.

The experience puts you right in the Patriots locker room, and then, later, lined up beside Tom Brady, in shotgun, as he calls a play. The ball is snapped, Brady drops back—and then fires a pass right by your ear, feeling real enough to make you duck.

A few seconds in STIVR is all I need to see how incredibly different—and how much better—this is than simply watching practice or game film. You're not watching from above; you've stepped *into* the film.

The only drawback is that STRIVR is not what experts call "true virtual reality." You can stand in the pocket beside Tom Brady or even as though you *are* Tom Brady, sure, and you can immerse yourself in a play as it unfolds—but you can't *play*. You are an observer, an invisible man in the middle of the action, but not a participant.

In true VR, you don't merely step into a world, you become *part* of it. You're not just standing beside Brady and watching him go to work. You become Tom Brady. You drop back. You make the reads. You make the calls. And you throw the ball.

That's not quite possible yet, but the company EON Sports is trying to get there.

EON SPORTS

As a freshman quarterback for Florida State in 2014, Jameis Winston led the Seminoles to a national title and, at nineteen years and 342 days old, became the youngest player to ever win the Heisman Trophy.

A year and a half later, when the Tampa Bay Buccaneers selected Winston as the first pick in the 2015 NFL Draft, they wanted to find something that would accelerate his transition into the NFL game, both in terms of their system and in adapting to the staggeringly faster speed of the men he'd be playing with and against now.

The Bucs called Brendan Reilly, the twenty-eight-year-old CEO of EON Sports, and asked him about the VR headsets—called the Sidekiq—on their website. Reilly sent them one. They loved it. Winston used it all the time. And he became that season's NFL Rookie of the Year.

Around the same time that Derek Belch was dreaming up ways that virtual reality could make the Stanford football team better prepared for games, Brendan Reilly, who is about Belch's age, was getting frustrated.

He wanted to be a college basketball coach. He was a student assistant for Bill Self at Kansas when the Jayhawks won the 2008 NCAA Championship. From there, he went to grad school at Illinois State, where he was a graduate assistant, and there, he started thinking a bit differently than everyone around him. "This was kind of around the time of the [publicizing] of the Moneyball era," he says. "Everyone was starting to find out about it—it was this really cool thing. And I just found statistics and technology in general, and the ways you could utilize both, kind of fascinating. I said, *If we're getting all this data, there's gotta be some way to visualize it, and that's gonna be really, really important to teams and their preparing of athletes.*"

He had no idea the direction technology would go from there. He just knew that he was spending hours upon hours splicing together game film, burning it to DVDs, and handing it out to athletes. "And," he says, "Lord knows if they watched two minutes of them, and I spent three hours making them. So it was a little bit born out of frustration. I was like, *Man, there's gotta be a better way to spend our time and train our athletes.*"

Part of Reilly's frustration was something he had learned while reading the book *Brain Rules* by Dr. John Medina; his big takeaway was a line saying, "There is no greater anti-brain environment than the classroom and the cubicle." Reilly says, "That's when I started going, *Okay, then what is? What's pro-brain?*"

Reilly started talking to people who worked in human performance. They told him that they used some virtual reality as part of simulated learning, and Reilly made an easy connection from what they were talking about to sports. "It just became very simple," he says.

If I understand him right, what became so very simple is the fact that the more someone does something and fails and then tries again, the more quickly they'll get good at it—but only if they do all of it in the actual environment they will be tested in, whether they are a surgeon or a basketball player trying to get better at shooting free throws. "You want to train *in* that environment," he says.

This is something I've come across often during this little knowledge quest. I've come to think of it as the Exposure Effect, and it's almost so commonsensical that we don't even need to get into the science of it. The idea is simple: the more you're exposed to something, the less intense it becomes, whether that intensity be adoration or terror or something else. This simply has to do with how much arousal the situation generates in the brain—by which I mean the scientific arousal, the activation of the brain. And this goes back to the insula, which helps predict the future.

An article in the January/February 2010 issue of *IEEE Computer Graphics and Applications* analyzes a gamut of various computer-based training regimens and film-study training for athletes, such as handball players. Its conclusion: "The next step is to develop the technology to create a virtual-sports training tool. By exploiting this immersive and interactive technology's advantages over video playback, coaches can put themselves in their players' shoes and experience what the player sees . . . video playback doesn't permit this type of in-depth analysis. Interactive, immersive virtual reality can overcome these limitations and foster a better understanding of sports performance."

All of this, combined with much of the research I've already covered, led Reilly to virtual reality. And there, he found sports leaders already saying that VR-like training regimens had immense potential. Inspired, he believed VR to be the next great leap in athletic training, and that, he says, led him to EON.

The company had been around for years, creating fantastic VR products that help with everything from engineering to aerospace to entertainment and all manner of education. They can let you go swimming with whales or put you in space, all from a comfy chair.

Reilly pestered the company, he says, for eighteen months. "I saw what they were already doing and I was like, 'You guys are sitting on a gold mine if you know how to leverage this for athletic training.'"

Eventually, sometime in 2009, they listened to him. They told him his idea was premature for the market, but they liked it. They offered him a job working on what they already had, and then they'd support him if he used his free time to work on sports.

As soon as Reilly joined EON, he realized his ambition for VR in sports was totally unrealistic. Laughing, he says, "The cost—I remember pitching, in my first meeting, the athletic directors at USC. And I'm sitting there, and I'm talking to them about the cost to do this, and it was just exorbitant. They all loved [the idea], but they were also like, 'We can't afford this! That's not something we can legitimately implement!' So that was a huge early barrier."

The technology was simply too expensive to make the move into sports.

But over the years, same as for STRIVR, tech caught up, and Reilly began to create.

Similar to STRIVR, the Sidekiq uses software that can put you in a 360-degree immersive video. But EON's other football software is fundamentally different in two ways. One, it looks and feels like a video game—something Reilly hypes, saying he puts people *in a Madden game.* Two, it's interactive. As the plays unfold, you have just a few seconds to make a decision about, say, where to throw the ball. You choose by moving your head until you're locked in on a receiver. It's like a blend of STRIVR and Axon, in a way, but where Axon gives you a good look at a team's defense, EON Sports has you playing against the defense itself. (You access its programs by downloading an app and then sticking your smartphone into the Sidekiq.)

EON custom-tailors what teams and players see according to their playbooks. It's not *quite* the same as watching real, live human beings running around out there, and you're not going to get all the variables you'd get in a practice or game, but the Sidekiq seems like an ideal supplement for an athlete's training.

It's already making an impact on big football names. There's Winston. Then there's Mike Ditka, the Hall of Fame former coach and current broadcaster who appears in Sidekiq promo videos, saying, "I started studying this game a long time ago, when I was a player, and then as an assistant coach under Coach Landry. And if Coach Landry and Coach Lombardi had this tool, it would've been so much easier to teach, and for the players to understand." Ditka goes on to say, "EON Sports is revolutionizing football in the way you study the game, in the way you understand your opponent, and the way you prepare for a football game."

Football is EON's flagship sport, but they've also made an ambitious foray into baseball.

EON Sports' marquee baseball program is Jason Giambi's Project OPS, hugely endorsed by Jason Giambi himself. In Project OPS, standing in the box, as you watch the pitches come in you also have to name the pitch and whether it was a ball or strike. You can use the Sidekiq, or play it like a video game on your smartphone. Giambi got turned on to EON by Dan O'Dowd, a former general manager for the Rockies who has served as EON and Reilly's adviser.

Reilly says that while it's great—not to mention lucrative—to build products that the elites can use, another big motivating factor is also envisioning how they will help young athletes, not only in football and baseball but eventually, he hopes, many other sports. EON is working on concepts for softball and cricket as well as basketball and soccer.

There's a feel-good aspect to this, to helping kids get better, but of course, it's also savvy business: in part because the youth levels don't need something quite as customizable and high end as the elites, which means it's way more scalable, and thus ultimately, potentially, far more profitable.

Project OPS, for instance, is primarily engineered as a strike-zone awareness app. When Reilly asked Giambi what he felt was one of the most underrated aspects of baseball training for young kids to develop, Giambi told him, "I watch kids today, and their strike-zone awareness is terrible. Kids just go up there and they don't even know why they're swinging at stuff. They just swing at it, or they just don't swing, like they decide before the pitch even to swing or not."

Giambi appears on the logo for the app and in the introductory videos, taking swings and showing you what you'll be doing. Even seems cool to me, an alleged grown-up. So yeah, for a kid? Out of this world.

EON isn't limited to headsets. You can play a little football or baseball by strapping on the Sidekiq, sure, but some teams are allowing their players to literally step into the virtual-reality world by taking the technology to the next level: Caves.

VR CAVES

Hidden deep in the training rooms of Major League Baseball stadiums around in the United States, there are huge technological cubes where the best ballplayers in the world take virtual batting practice. The cubes are composed of walls upon which a computer program is projected. The ballplayer puts on glasses that bring the projections into focus, at which point he finds himself standing in a batter's box, facing a big-league pitcher.

EON builds these cubes. The details are, of course, top secret. But if those big-league cubes are anything like the simulator EON Sports set up at the 2016 Consumer Electronics Show, then we can have a pretty good idea.

Industry lingo for these cubes is *CAVE*. That stands for "cave automatic virtual environment." The first VR cave ever created was in 1991, and it was outlandishly expensive. The MLB caves cost hundreds of thousands of dollars. The EON CAVE at CES was a bit less intense, ten feet by ten feet by ten feet, with the front wall and the floor being screens. (In the full versions, the side walls are also screens.)

Troy Tulowitzki from the Rockies (now the Jays) even stopped by and declared, "It's pretty real."

Step one: put on the motion-tracking stereoscopic LCD shutter glasses. They will not only bring the projections into focus, but they have three sensors on each frame—two projectors control the system, with two motion-capture cameras coupled with the glasses' sensors, shifting the VR environment as you move.

Step two: kick off your shoes and/or slip on some slippers.

Step three: take the bat, which is basically a regular bat with sensors on it, step into the cave, and take your stance in the batter's box.

Step four: try to hit the digital baseballs the digital pitcher is throwing you. Fastballs, curveballs, change-ups. A setting in the program can show you, in the top left of the screen in front of you, what the pitcher is about to throw—or not. The pitchers can throw everything from 83-mph curve balls to 96-mph fastballs, and the like. Real big-league stuff, if you want. Coaches can even control what pitch is thrown and where it goes.

That's the advantage of his system. It's not really going to be batting practice as much as an über-immersive way to see some live pitches without actually facing live pitching. Batting practice is swing refining and confidence building, but live pitching is another beast, and the EON CAVE is a truly sci-fi hitting supplement, like a pitching machine come to life.

Getting comfortable with live pitching is one of every ballplayer's greatest struggles at the beginning of any season. Sometimes I'd watch video of old games and try to imagine facing the pitcher live, but obviously that's nothing compared to these beautiful technological beasts. You stand in a virtual batter's box in front of a virtual pitcher and get to see real pitches thrown at you. Even if you're not "really" swinging and hitting them, just getting to *see* them is incredible.

Between the apps, the Sidekiq, and the CAVE concept, Reilly likes to sell EON Sports' baseball offerings as, "You get to play against Clayton Kershaw before you actually play Clayton Kershaw," referring to the Los Angeles Dodgers pitcher who's won the National League Cy Young Award three times.

Let me be perfectly clear: this isn't *quite* like facing Kershaw. EON Sports' offerings are still video games, nothing more or less: you're not literally seeing Clayton Kershaw's specific pitches.

That said, you get a pretty good idea. Far beyond better than not doing it. And it's not easy. Or maybe I just suck worse than I thought. All I know is, I had a hard time with it for a little while, until I got the hang of it.

Reilly has his top-tier customers, including three Major League teams for whom he's built CAVEs in their training facilities. Over the years, as with all technology, the EON Sports CAVE will only become more affordable, and Reilly will be able to make more sales. "It's a lot easier now," he says. "People get what it is, they have a good idea of why this can add value, so the old days of being met with silence on the other end of the phone . . . those days are long gone."

As Reilly developed the EON CAVE concept he drew a lot of inspiration from the Duke Immersive Virtual Environment (DiVE) at Duke University. He went to Duke and met with the folks that run the DiVE, and he was, after a venture into the DiVE itself, left with a sense of wonder. He says, "That's, like, the Taj Mahal."

THE TAJ MAHAL OF VIRTUAL REALITY

Stepping into the DiVE feels like a taste of the Matrix. Thankfully, you don't have to plug your skull into a computer, but once in that cave, you quickly lose any sense of place beyond what the cave provides.

I get invited to check it out by Dr. Greg Appelbaum. You know his name by now. Among many other things, Appelbaum studies the impact of vision on the cognitive performance of athletes. The DiVE proves most useful.

In room 1617A on the first floor of the CIEMAS (Fitzpatrick Center), in the Engineering Quad on West Campus, the DiVE began operation in 2006 and was just the fourth six-sided CAVE-like system in the United States.

Appelbaum walks me over and introduces me to DiVE research and development engineer David Zielinski, a very nice, excited guy in this thirties.

After we talk, I go in. I pull some black slippers over my shoes and put on the glasses. When I step in, the wall slides shut behind me.

Then the only world I know is the world DiVE shows me.

Well, DiVE and Zielinski. He's in here, too, holding a remote that he uses to manipulate the environment.

Where EON's CAVEs, such as the one I saw at CES 2016, are generally one-story constructions within a relatively confined space—again, ten-by-ten-by-ten with a few sensors, projectors, and cameras—Duke's DiVE spans three floors and consumes an entire laboratory. The EON Sports CAVE at the CES on steroids. There's even a viewing area behind a large glass window, and when prospective students are given campus tours, they'll often stare in at the DiVE and the engineers running it, their mouths dropping open. "Yeah," Zielinski says, "I feel like I'm in a zoo sometimes."

Once we're closed in, Zielinski cues up an earthy, wilderness-like world that is somewhat pixelated, reminding me of Minecraft or old video games.

"Turn around, check it out," he says.

I turn, and there's a woman walking toward me; she stops right beside me. She is, of course, also distinctly video-game-y, but she feels *real*, especially as she's staring at me. Video-game character or not, it's freaky. "If feels like there's a person right there," I say.

"Yeah, it's not like we're looking at a screen or 3-D movie or anything," Zielinski says. "All right. Now let's see where she goes."

She walks past me and toward a cliff with a bridge that connects it to another, distant cliff—but she misses the bridge and drops off the edge.

I know it's a simulation, and yet my heart still bursts seeing someone—"someone"—drop like that.

"Let's go take a look," Zielinski says.

The simulation transports us onto the bridge, and now I'm staring down a thousand-foot drop. My knees go weak and I start sweating. Feeling dumb and amazed and laughing, I say, "Dude, I feel like I'm about to fall!"

Zielinski grins, and then that's exactly what we're doing, falling a thousand feet. I kid you not, without even thinking, I bend my knees, catching balance after a fall that never actually happened, and for a brief moment there, I'm worried I might crap myself. When we land—"land"—I feel a very real sense of relief.

And then, when I start to say something, I realize I'm out of breath somehow. "Dude, it feels so *real*."

So, what does all this have to do with sports?

That brings us to Appelbaum.

In one of his recent experiments he had a dozen volunteers strap an EEG cap to their heads, hook into a computer, and then grab a gun. Well, grab Zielinski's remote, to be specific. It has a vaguely gunlike design and doubles as a virtual pistol/shotgun/whatever might be needed. (They're working on getting replicas to use with the DiVE.)

Appelbaum loaded a clay-shooting program, and the test subjects shot the clays, same as at any competitive shooting event. He used the EEG to collect data on when the subjects made decisions and how long it took, etc.

All of this to say, he's working on acquiring grant money to bring in members of the U.S. Olympic shooting team in order to study them and help them train in a new way. And that's only going to be the start. He's simmering with all sorts of ideas, hoping to build until he can design programs that work with all kinds of athletes.

When I was a kid, maybe eight years old, my class took a field trip to the Imagination Station Science Museum in Wilson, North Carolina. By far the coolest thing there for us little dudes and dudettes was this simulator that let us "race" animals. Turtles, horses, cheetahs. We'd choose our opponent, wait for a countdown, and then sprint like all heck, racing the "animal" by racing streaking light on the wall beside us.

I can't help but imagine some similar sensational combination of headsets and CAVE systems, massive simulators the size of gyms. We can get in the box and *really* face Clayton Kershaw, or line up *as* Tom Brady, or get in defensive position with LeBron James dribbling downcourt. Us against their holograms.

The implications of such systems for athletes are enormous, especially as all of the technology keeps developing. The headset software, the EON CAVEs, even Duke's DiVE, like so much of This Stuff, seem so mind-blowing and cutting edge right now— and yet the more I learn, the more apparent it becomes that really, while the systems are exciting because they are, in many ways, brand-new, they are also kind of *brand-new.* In their infancy, really. Barring some sort of apocalyptic solar storm frying all our tech, someday in the near future, the worlds where athletes live and the worlds wherein they train may hardly be distinguishable one from the other. (Who knows—in the future, we might not need real athletes at all.)

Regardless of how innovative your training, and how neurocognitively efficient your methods, and how cutting edge your tech, and how brain-train-y your brain training, all of it can be rendered useless by one thing, something that we often think of as *outside* the brain, although it really flows *through* the brain: vision.

Chapter 16

Window to the Brain

Steph Curry dribbles a basketball with one hand and with his other tosses a tennis ball back and forth with his trainer. This is just one in a long series of his typical, elaborate dribbling drills— only he's also wearing some sort of goggles, the lenses of which seem to be flashing black.

I saw this in a video that went viral in late fall 2015, and it leads me back to Oliver Marmol, the St. Louis Cardinals coach we met earlier.

Those goggles are his product, created in partnership with a company called Sensory Performance Technology. He calls them the Eclipse. Curry uses them through all kinds of different drills; they're one of his trainer Brandon Payne's favorites for *enhancing neurocognitive efficiency.*

As Marmol "got into the neuro side of things," around 2011, he started some experimental training with his players using Nike's Vapor Strobe goggles—their lenses flash at various speeds to obscure the vision. Marmol saw some remarkable results, the most profound of which occurred for one of his baseball players, whom we'll call Biff.

Marmol drilled Biff using the strobes fifteen minutes a day six days a week for about six weeks. Marmol started by blocking 10 percent of Biff's eyesight while he was hitting off a pitching machine throwing 85 mph. They worked up to 20, 30, 40 percent until Biff was doing well, then cranked it up to 90 mph and reduced the occlusion—the blocking of information—back to 10 percent, then worked their way back up to 40 percent again at 90 mph. Then they went to 95 and repeated. They also worked with contrast sensitivity, using different-colored balls to hit and such, but the strobes played an integral role.

Biff improved his batting average from .122 to .286, and he went from striking out every other at-bat to going four or five at-bats between strikeouts. "Some of the craziest gains," Marmol says.

It's all the same idea as weight lifting, cardio, any kind of physical training: overload your system until you adapt, until you become stronger, rinse, repeat. Marmol says, "I want the guys I'm training to be really struggling through exercises, where they're having to tap into the same mental state that they're going to experience in a game. That's where true growth actually happens . . . And as we continue to pump out research and do what we're doing, I think we're going to see some incredible things in the sporting world."

Marmol partnered with Sensory Performance Technology to develop and sell the Eclipse as an updated version of the Vapor Strobes after Nike discontinued the product a few years ago.

However, he has stiff competition from another company started by the very man who helped create the Nike Vapor Strobes in the first place.

In an office in a business park in Beaverton, Oregon, just around the corner from Nike World Headquarters, I'm standing in front of a huge touch-screen monitor wearing strobe goggles, poking—rapidly, violently poking—neon circles that flash onto the screen, while also reading strings of numbers eight digits long, *and* Herb Yoo is shoving me. Every second or so, for a split second, the goggle lenses turn completely gray and that's all I can see. Because of this, I'm having a hard time keeping my balance—and *now* Yoo's throwing a ball for me to catch, and I'm still trying to read the numbers and poke the screen, and I almost fall over, and I definitely don't catch the ball.

Now Yoo's laughing at me, and so is his business partner, Joe Bingold, from the next room over, where he's playing with a fifteen-foot-long electric snake hooked up to his computer and flashing different colors.

Yoo and Bingold are two of the founders of Senaptec, a company built around the big touch screen I'm training on—the Sensory Station—as well as their other flagship product, the goggles I'm wearing, called Strobes. They have a saying: *the eyes are the window to the brain.* And their whole idea is to build better vision by building a stronger brain.

This brings us to one of the most stunning things I've learned so far. We have five senses, right? We experience those senses because of specialized cells throughout our body called *sensory receptors.* Everything you feel, hear, smell, taste, and see comes from those receptors sending the information they gather to your brain.

Of all the sensory receptors we have, 70 percent are in our eyes alone.

That's 260 million (130 mil per eye) receptors taking information in through the eyes and sending it to the brain, by way of 2.4

million nerve fibers. This adds up to our eyes sending our brain 109 gigabytes of data *every second.*

Sidenote: Red Bull's Andy Walshe tells me, "There's an augmentation conversation in the pipeline, which is not Red Bull, but in the greatest context of human performance, *hey, let's make everybody twenty/ten, with Lasik or restorative contacts.* Which hey, why not? There's no rules against it now."

But first, someone has to realize they need augmentation, whether Lasik or simply through training. In a sense, that is Senaptec's role. Not that they tell people to get Lasik, but they have cutting-edge means by which to help people understand and improve their vision. Yoo, the Senaptec CTO, says, "Even the practitioners in the high-performance world will acknowledge that the sensory cognition, that neuro, is the new frontier. You have to know the world before you can act upon it."

If Senaptec sounds vaguely familiar, here's why: a few years ago, Nike created its SPARQ Sensory Performance division, which included, you guessed it, a Sensory Station and Strobe goggles. Yoo was the director of innovation at Nike at the time, and he was one of the primary guys working on the SPARQ brand. It was his dream job. He's from Beaverton, so he was working in his hometown, at the world headquarters of one of the world's most dynamic businesses. He could explore virtually whatever he wanted.

And on top of all that, he was working directly with some of the world's most famous athletes, in ways nobody else at the company could match. "That was the only way to know how to help them," Yoo says. A pleasant person, Yoo often speaks with a little grin on his face, giddy. "We'd have to go to their practices or their facilities and see, okay, how are you working, what are you doing, and what can we do to make you better?"

The idea behind the Sensory Station was to create a battery

of tests for athletes' vision. The development of the Strobes was based in large part on a scientific study done on athletes training in a dark room with a strobe light turned on.

The SPARQ project moved along well. Nike launched the SPARQ Sensory Performance Station and the SPARQ Vapor Strobes in the fall of 2011, to critical acclaim. They created a dedicated server on which all of the data from their Sensory Station was stored, allowing athletes to anonymously compare themselves with their peers. They got dozens of pro teams interested, selling them units for prices well into five figures, and the Vapor Strobes were being researched by neuroscientists with excellent results. "Sensory Training Technology Takes Hold in the NFL," declared *Time* magazine in January 2012. "Nike's SPARQ Shines a Light on Visual Training," a *Wired* magazine headline raved that February.

And then suddenly, in late 2013, Nike shut down the whole Sensory Performance division.

Nike's official story—and the story Yoo tells me—is that the higher-ups apparently felt like they were getting too far afield and wanted to refocus on their core business, which is footwear and apparel, so they abruptly pulled the plug on SPARQ.

The move left Herb Yoo and his colleagues stunned. "We had so much research and we had made such great progress," Yoo says. "We felt like it was a shame to just let it all go for nothing."

One of Yoo's primary supporters was Pete Naschak, a former Navy SEAL turned leadership expert who consults with Nike, Red Bull, and several other companies. He'd been involved in the Sensory Performance projects, and encouraged Yoo to try doing something more with it. Yoo also reached out to a few others who had been doing research with the SPARQ products, such as Dr. Jason Mihalik at UNC–Chapel Hill, who'd been using them in his concussion research, to see if they'd be interested. They were.

Naschak is now the Senaptec COO, and Mihalik the chief science officer.

Yoo also asked Joe Bingold, a friend from his church, if he'd be interested in helping him start a company to continue producing this stuff because, frankly, he felt he could make it better. Bingold is now their CEO. He triple-majored at MIT and spent eight years in the Navy working on the Nuclear Propulsion Program, largely responsible for the nuclear-power electronic control systems on aircraft carriers and submarines. After that, he got his MBA at the Stanford Graduate School of Business, then cofounded another start-up and worked as director of marketing for Tektronix. He's an ambitious guy, and he liked Yoo's concepts. Plus, Bingold saw this as something that could make the world a better place, and, he says, "Sorry, I'm a sucker—I'm a romantic."

They were taking an enormous risk. Both Yoo and Bingold have wives and two kids, and they were used to high-paying executive salaries. This move sent them into start-up mode.

But it was a risk worth taking because when Bingold looked at what Yoo wanted to do, he saw a way to change the world. "This is really the next phase of human performance," he says. "It's sort of this untapped area. We all assume we see the same, hear the same, and everything like that, but we don't. And being able to assess and improve is pretty cool. And for me, sports is one thing, but then brain health and mental health and all that, and where that could go, is really exciting, because really, it could help people who don't have tools to get better."

Helping lessen the risk was the fact that, after some doing, Yoo and his new team convinced Nike to license their Sensory Performance products' technology, using that to launch what is now Senaptec. (They're probably having a fit right now as they read this, by the way, because part of their agreement with Nike was to never tell anyone about said licensing. So let me be clear: Yoo and his colleagues didn't spill the beans, Nike. Some other folks filled me in.)

That was two years ago.

Now Senaptec has sold a couple dozen of their units to everyone from pro sports teams to the military, including the New York Yankees and various Red Bull athletes. Red Bull installed their Senaptec station right beside several other brain enhancement technologies and right behind some weight racks. Andy Walshe is fired up about it. "[It's] a really good test of vision that's fun," he says. "There's a dynamic vision test in this . . . All that's really helpful. We could do a standard test, 'stare at an eye chart,' like they do at the DMV. And that would be helpful. But this is the twenty-first-century version of that."

Senaptec remains very much a start-up. The office suite where I meet Yoo and Bingold—number 195 at 3800 Cedar Hills Boulevard in Beaverton—isn't even all theirs. They share a lobby and conference room with a few other companies in the same suite, and they have a single small office to call their own. They won it in a local start-up competition.

Yoo answers the door when I arrive. He and Bingold both wear khakis, casual loafers, and patterned shirts, tucked in, with clean-cut dark hair parted neatly on the side. Herb has a laid-back demeanor while Joe has the sharp eyes of a business shark; they're both eager to talk.

And in one of their offices is one of their other two babies, the Senaptec Sensory Station. It looks like a fifty-inch flat-screen television mounted on a thick, strong stand anchored to a sturdy base with wheels. The screen can be raised or lowered according to the user's eye level, and it's made of tempered glass so that you can really poke the heck out of it when going through the exercises without fear of breaking it.

One of the first things I ask them is *Why?* Despite licensing the

Nike tech, what drives someone to leave a dream job (and salary) as a Nike executive to jump into start-up mode?

Yoo says, "It came down to, you know, *What's the mission?*"

He didn't want to go back to the footwear world. Not after seeing what he and a good team of scientific minds could create. Even the realists at Nike know that the shoes you wear don't matter *that* much.

Plus, people were still using what he'd help create, both in sports and in the military. "It wasn't like this was going to get completely shut off immediately," Yoo says. And he knew that more research was in the pipeline—DARPA (the Defense Advanced Research Projects Agency) had just funded a million-dollar study to look at how much the Sensory Station and Strobes could help soldiers. Yoo says, "There's going to be a lot of . . . research that's going to be publicly available, things to stand on to say, 'I helped develop this technology, I helped set up these research partnerships, to get some independent findings out there.'"

Moreover, Yoo knew how crucial good vision was. Arsène Wenger, the legendary manager of the Arsenal soccer club in Europe, once told him, "The single most important skill on the pitch is peripheral vision."

Yoo says, "He didn't talk about any physical skills. He's talking about a sensory visual skill."

It makes perfect sense when you think about it: of *course* vision's the most important aspect of sports. There's no major sport in the world you could imagine someone playing well with impaired vision. And yet how often do people talk about vision, and how to enhance it? Yoo says, "You may have heard coaches, or analysts in the media, say, 'Oh, *that athlete has great vision.*' But what does that really mean? They don't know. They're using the term *vision* as this umbrella term. But if we can start to break it down, we can pinpoint—better athletes have better visual skills."

Wayne Gretzky, Yoo points out, famously said that he skates where the puck will be, not where it is. Larry Fitzgerald, the great Arizona Cardinals wide receiver, did vision training as a child with his grandfather, an optometrist. "Parents need to understand," Fitzgerald once said, "that you need over 17 visual skills to succeed. Seeing 20/20 is just one of those. Vision problems can have a serious impact." And not just in sports, he added, but also "on a child's education."

Then there's Babe Ruth. In 1921, researchers from Columbia University's psychology department performed some studies on the Great Bambino, and they found that he had one of the most remarkable sets of eyes and athletic brains in existence at the time. He processed visual information 12 percent faster than normal men, and compared to the normal man, Babe's visual perception occurred 150 percent faster.

Yoo takes me out into the lobby, where we toss a Wiffle ball. "Okay, so you're pretty good at this," he says after I catch it and lob it back a couple times. "I mean, you have your other hand in your pocket, right?"

Um, indeed.

"Okay, now put these on." He hands me a pair of the Strobes, turning them on level two. The goggles are comfortable, easily wrapping around my eyes and held in place by a comfortable strap—remember Rec Specs? I don't think anyone wears them anymore, but back in the day, they were what athletes needing prescription eyewear wore. Big, bulky, dorky looking, strapped in place by a band around the back of the head. The Strobes are kind of like that, except sleek and athletic in design, with a modern, even space-age-y feel.

The lenses are made from liquid crystal, and unlike their first iteration as Nike's SPARQ Vapor Strobes, the Senaptec Strobes are waterproof and can be segmented, blocking out portions of the lenses instead of the whole thing.

The lenses flashing, Yoo throws at me again. A little tougher, but still not too bad.

We keep increasing the level, the Strobes flashing more often and staying dark longer at a time. Soon I'm fumbling after the ball and running into stuff and sweating.

After about ten minutes of this, when I pull the goggles off, I feel dizzy and a little seasick. "That is *intense,*" I say, laughing with Yoo and Bingold, who sat there watching and poking fun at me the whole time.

Yoo tosses me the ball again, and nothing in the world has ever felt easier—and more of a *relief*—than simply being able to see something thrown at me and catching it.

It's easy to see vast applications for the Strobes. They are perfect for blocking drills as a catcher and for taking a little soft toss or batting practice as a hitter. You can extrapolate that across tons of sports. The most common feedback they get is, "This slows the game down."

There was a study a couple years ago examining how much the Strobes helped athletes, using the Carolina Hurricanes hockey team in Raleigh, North Carolina. The results were so stunning that scientific journals have been rejecting the study because their editors don't believe them. Performed over three weeks from August to September 2011, using the Nike Sparq Vapor Strobes, the study showed that training with the goggles improved vision, attention, and anticipatory timing. The researchers had eleven players participate, seven forwards and four defensemen. Names were drawn to determine the Strobe group and the control group. Six of the players ending up using Strobes. They were then put through a variety of drills, and scored on things like how well they shot after skating a certain pattern, making long passes, and the like.

By the end of the study, the control group remained the same—they actually went down 2 percent as a group—while the guys in the Strobe group improved 11 to 29 percent, with an average of 18 percent.

Another study in 2011 used the Strobes to test a group of students at Southern Utah State, putting them through a series of tests on an anticipatory timing device commonly used in scientific experiments. The results found that training with the Strobes improved anticipatory timing after training.

In 2011, Appelbaum (along with some other researchers) even found that training with Strobes improved people's short-term memory.

A 2012 study, performed with sixteen members of the Utah State University football team, tested whether an athlete could use the Strobes to improve what's known in the science world as "dynamic visual acuity"—that is, how well you can recognize and track a moving object while you are also moving. It's an important athletic skill—a wide receiver turning to see the ball headed right for him, a hockey player finding a puck passed to him, a basketball player catching a sudden pass. The study found that training with the Strobes improved players' ability to react to moving objects while moving themselves.

Yoo once worked with an ice hockey trainer who lost vision in one of his eyes after getting hit with a puck. After training with the Strobes for fifteen minutes, he came back to Yoo and said that he felt like he'd gotten both of his eyes back.

Then there's the Sensory Station. It can be used in combination with the Strobes, though more often it is not. The Sensory Station measures and trains about a dozen different visual and "sensorimotor" skills, such as visual clarity (how well you pick up details, such as the spin on a baseball), contrast sensitivity (how well you differentiate between, say, a baseball and a cloud), depth perception, near-far quickness (how quickly you can shift your attention from near objects to far ones), perception span (how quickly you visually acquire critical information), reaction time, multiple object tracking, target capture (how quickly you find and take action against a peripheral target), eye-hand coordination (this is the flashing-dots part I was talking about earlier; when lights appear, you press them, measuring how quickly you can respond to changing targets), and Go/No Go (the same idea as eye-hand coordination, except not pressing the lights when they're red instead of green).

The whole process only takes about half an hour. By the end of it, not only do athletes know if they have twenty-twenty vision or better, but they're also shown how strong they are in matters of vision that go beyond mere eyesight into how well their brain is processing what their eyes see: how well they pay attention, how quickly they respond to changes in their surroundings, how well they handle stress, how strong their impulse control is, and so on.

Better yet, as soon as their analysis is finished, Senaptec instantly generates a results map, a circular grid identifying where the athlete stands compared to her peers. And from that, Senaptec also instantly creates a recommended training program.

Then, also using the Senaptec Station, the athletes can begin training immediately. The training programs change in appearance from the assessments, and are intuitive, shifting in difficulty according to performance, pushing the athlete without becoming overwhelming.

It's easy to see why Yoo and Bingold and the others got on this start-up train. Senaptec is still brand-new, but in terms of tech, science, and experience, the company's work might be the one aspect of This Stuff that I'd be shocked to see not catch on and become part of every elite and aspiring elite athletes' training. It feels nothing like a visit to the eye doctor, yet checks all the same things and more.

Its potential goes beyond improving vision and attention and all those other important sports things—the Sensory Station could also end up having dramatic impact on the medical side, too.

Jason Mihalik at UNC is using it for concussion work. "It can be a wonderful baseline tool," he says, meaning that it's great for testing athletes before seasons begin, so that if they suffer a head injury he can test them again and see where their weaknesses are, thus discovering where they perhaps suffered greatest injury—discovering as well how to best help them rehab. And then he can use the Sensory Station's training tools as part of the rehab.

Yoo says that they're still waiting on the results of some studies, but it's feasible to think that the tech could also help stroke victims, children with ADHD, and other mental health concerns.

He says, "What's exciting is being able to find a way to help someone to get better, [a way] that's legal, and that [people] haven't even tried before. There's acceleration training, there's speed training, there's plyometrics—a lot of options in the physical space. Practitioners would say they've been maxed out. What's really needed is something new in the space to help athletes. And I say athletes—could be combat athletes or sport athletes. And in the long term, it's helping those like we talked about before— below the normal range—to get back into their quote 'normal' lifestyle."

Halfway around the world, the concepts of Senaptec are taking hold, already generating fantastic results.

Erez Morag worked at Nike in Beaverton for more than a decade as a lead researcher responsible for ensuring that the company—one of the most innovative in the world—kept innovating. To innovate is to see the future, and when Morag looked into the future, he saw cognitive training. He became so passionate about it that, in 2011, he moved back to his beloved home country, Israel, to start his own cog-training company, Innov8,

with a sports division, Acceler8, in a laboratory not far from Je-
rusalem.

Morag's mission, in his words: "To enhance speed of thoughts
in sports with the use of advanced technologies." Among his primary technologies was the Sensory Station. "The way I define my
job, I am a translator," he says. "I translate science into action."

However, Morag knew "implementing new methodologies in
training is often a challenge." Thus, he first sought out forward-
thinking, visionary coaches who were open to new ideas.

The first coach to visit Morag's lab was David Blatt, who, before coming to the United States to coach the Cleveland Cavaliers,
coached Israel's Maccabi Tel Aviv and won several championships,
a dynasty in their own right. Morag remembers Blatt quoting his
former coach at Princeton, the legendary Hall of Famer Pete Car-
ril, who used to choose players based on one key criterion: "Can
they see?"

Morag began working with Blatt and Maccabi, and some others. He was primarily focused on soccer, basketball, and tennis.

And, he says, "The results I've seen are amazing. Absolutely
amazing. This is such untapped territory."

Among those results of which Morag speaks there is one particular story that to the casual—or, let's face it, even devout—fan
is out of left field, yet as inspiring as any great sports movie.

One of the first coaches to visit his lab was, Morag says, quite
a surprise: Ira Vigdorchik, head coach for the Israeli National
Rhythmic Gymnastics Team.

Vigdorchik wanted to take their young, promising team into
the final quarter of their season with a major goal in mind: winning
the world championships in September. Morag describes Vigdorchik as "a fast thinker" and "highly respected in her field," and
says that she "felt that cognitive training [could] help her team prepare for the event."

One of the team's main events was called the "10 Clubs Competition." "Highly challenging," Morag says. Five girls, each holding two batonlike clubs, perform a coordinated gymnastic routine to music for two and a half minutes, including lots of throwing and catching in highly challenging positions.

The young team had found success at the juniors level, but Vigdorchik wanted to make them perform better, especially under pressure, and perhaps most importantly, cut down on their number of drops.

She felt that the best way to do that was through specific cognitive training.

Morag's methods, he keeps mostly to himself, but in general, he says, "I believe in simplicity." He's using virtually the same tech as Senaptec, only perhaps a bit older. He assesses much of the same visual skills, his goal being to help determine athletes' abilities to see their game, process information, and react quickly and accurately to what's happening. Then he'll take them out of the lab and onto the training field next door and they'll work. Then, after some training, they return to the lab and take a second assessment. Based on that assessment, he prescribes more training.

Morag followed that routine with the gymnasts and in his on-field training incorporated the use of the stroboscopic goggles. "The rationale," he says, "was to take away part of the visual information when training in order to develop better anticipation, eye-hand coordination, and choice reaction time. These qualities can translate to better throwing and catching of the clubs, better chances to 'save' and catch a bad throw, and better sync between athletes."

They had the same goal as any athletic competitor—to win—but let's be honest, their expectations weren't very high. They were a new, young team going against the best in the world. They knew their odds; they truly just wanted to compete. And compete they did, finishing fifth in the overall competition. However, they shocked the rhythmic gymnastics world in their Ten Clubs Competition.

Over the two-day event, they were the only team in the world to not drop a single club—and they took home a silver medal, finishing even ahead of Russia, an outcome Morag exuberantly equates with Team USA beating Russia in hockey in the 1980 Olympics. A very David-versus-Goliath win, unlikely and beautiful.

PART FOUR

THE SPIRIT

In so many unspoken ways, masterful performance isn't about performance at all; instead it's about what resides within us and drives us to perform. I found athletes doing breathtaking things in pursuit of a better spirit, and remarkable stories behind what those things do for them, and how those things even came to exist in the first place.

Despite all that modern science is teaching us and helping us to create in order to make the most out of our minds, there are also mind-bending methods being used around the world to strengthen the spirit—even as, in some ways, they transcend science.

With sports serving as my metaphor for careers and dreams and other goals—for all the things that really matter to us in our lives—I felt compelled to pursue them.

Sometimes, no amount of sport-specific training can do anything to ease the anxiety, or fear, or depression, or whatever other monsters keep messing with you. That's the bad news. The good news is that there are still things you can do.

Sometimes, dealing with matters of the soul means doing simple things. Talking with a therapist or counselor: *Great*. Meditation: *Great*. Gratitude journal: *Great*. There is neuroscience to back up all of this and more. Gratitude, for instance, boosts dopamine and serotonin, and it has been found to be as good for mental health, in some cases, as antidepressants. When we consciously think about something we are grateful for, it makes the brain react as though we just received a gift or reward. USC Shoah Foundation executive director Dr. Stephen D. Smith once said that Holocaust survivors told the foundation that when someone did something nice for them during their terrible times, such as giving them some food or providing a place to hide, the gratitude that they felt "helped them hold on to their humanity."

Gratitude has also been shown in studies to increase determination, attention, enthusiasm, and energy. When one of his players was struggling after a bad game, Urban Meyer texted back and forth with him every morning for weeks to talk about the things they were grateful for, which helped the young man tremendously.

Studies have also shown that gratitude spirals beyond a single grateful brain—the more grateful one person is, the more they are compelled to do things that make other people feel grateful, too. It's all a virus, in a way. Sometimes, the virus can be good for us.

Likewise, holding a grudge floods our brains with cortisol, known as "the stress hormone," which is generated when our *homeostasis* veers off course in favor of the sympathetic nervous system, activating our fight-or-flight response. At the same time, cortisol drains us of oxytocin, the feel-good neurotransmitter, which balances such stress.

In the 1970s, a surgeon and burn specialist, Dr. Dabney Ewin, discovered that as he worked with burn victims not only on their physical healing, but also on letting go of anger and finding forgiveness, their wounds healed faster. Some patients who would typically need months to heal—and with multiple skin grafts and sometimes amputations—were healing within two or three weeks, without so much as a single skin graft.

Patients who remained angry, on the other hand, required multiple skin grafts that their body would then often reject. Ewin realized, as he told his patients, "What you're feeling will affect the healing of your skin, and we want you to put all your energy into healing." If you resolve the conflict or let go of the anger, the cortisol drains away while the oxytocin floods back in.

And sometimes, cortisol and oxytocin can work together to create *eustress,* a term for the "good" stress we experience when we are feeling passion and purpose. (The opposite of that is called a much more familiar word, *distress,* the origin of which has to do with disease.)

This is especially important for teammates, whether players or coaches or otherwise. Not only is a cortisol imbalance poison for the brain, but too little oxytocin can harm the brain's ability to process information, which means that if teammates are feuding off the court, it can very literally affect how they play on the court.

Ditto if something goes wrong on the court. Compassion works in a similar way.

Dr. Robert Enright, a developmental psychologist at the University of Wisconsin–Madison, conducted a study in 2008 that explored the differences between two groups of people suffering from coronary heart disease. One group received standard medical care, reminders to eat right and exercise, and so on. Another group received "forgiveness therapy." The group who learned how to forgive became healthier, specifically by receiving more blood flow to their hearts.

Of course, all of these issues and more can be managed through talk therapy with the Mike Gervaises of the world.

As I went deeper and deeper down this rabbit hole, however, I ended up with what you'll find in this section, where athletes are taking the notion of bettering their spirit to its fullest extreme. I want the most out of my mind? I want my mind truly strong, truly right? I have to be willing to go everywhere, even the darkest, strangest places, both literally and figuratively. Just when I think I've learned all I can, I'll find that there's always something more to learn.

That's what this is all about in a way, though, right?

No matter how much I *know*, no matter how much I learn about myself, no matter how much I grow as a person, sometimes I need to just do something that stretches me beyond myself, for reasons I can't explain going into it, reasons I might not understand until afterward.

That's what the people you're about to meet have shown me.

For this last section, we'll settle into a few good stories, because good stories are hard to beat when it comes to finding the best way to strengthen the spirit.

And if you thought where we've been so far has been intense or strange, well, buckle up.

Chapter 17

Project Acheron

In Dante's *Inferno,* the border to Hell is formed by the River Acheron (pronounced "ACK-er-on"), also known as the River of Pain. That's where Red Bull's Project Acheron gets its name.

Project Acheron is an expedition series designed to push athletes to their limits, in every sense. The idea came to Andy Walshe in a fit of inspiration fueled by the philosophy of the ancient Shaolin fighting monks and Japanese samurai. They became so masterful with the sword that, Walshe says, "They spent more time working on inner spirit. They picked these arduous challenges every two or three years, to see what they're made of—to find the limits to their souls. I said to myself, *Why can't we re-create that with a modern twist?* Let's take that ancient idea of using a spiritual, physical challenge to find out what you're made of, and use that to become more masterful in your chosen craft."

Project Acheron began in early 2014, with big-wave surfer Ian Walsh, kayaker Rafa Ortiz, Surf Ironman champ Matt Poole, and waterman Kai Lenny.

Walshe's vision was to take athletes where no one had ever gone before, and not just figuratively: one of their destinations—unbeknownst to the guys—was to summit a Patagonian mountain peak nobody else had ever climbed. His reasoning is straightforward: "When you're at the pinnacle of your sport, the only way to progress is to move beyond that comfort zone."

Of all the guys, Walshe expected Acheron to be most beneficial for Lenny, a champion in standup paddle boarding and kite surfing and a renowned young big-wave surfer. He was basically still a kid at the time, a mere twenty years old, and only beginning to step into the senior ranks of his sports, clearly the most boyish of the four. Walshe thought Acheron would turn him into a man.

The guys were dropped off in the middle of nowhere in the middle of the night in Patagonia, Chile. None of them knew what they were getting into. And the truth was *nobody,* at Red Bull or otherwise, fully knew just how extreme the excursion would become. Walshe designed it with Pete Naschak, the retired Navy SEAL turned leadership coach, who would serve as expedition leader, with input from Steve Sanders, also a retired SEAL, along with a spiritual adviser and a veteran Patagonian mountain guide. The designers had *some* idea of how tough it would be, but a lot of it was also guesswork—a massive experiment, really.

Before the guys set off for Chile, they went to the University of California–San Diego. There, they received what Walshe calls "one of the most comprehensive work-ups of any athlete group I've ever seen." Walshe wanted a baseline to compare the guys against two weeks later, when they returned. Physical assessments, sure—nutrition panels, blood DNA markers, gut biome analyses—but also psychiatric exams conducted by professor of psychiatry Dr. Martin Paulus.

One of Walshe's goals with Project Acheron was to see how undertaking a spiritual quest might change the brain, particularly its perception of stress and its reaction to it. To that end, a significant part of the Paulus examination involved an EEG assessment and fMRI scans.

Paulus was downright giddy. He'd never worked on anything like Project Acheron. Lots of other studies, sure, but with Acheron, he told Walshe, "you have basically a brain scan before you expose the person to a certain type of challenge, and then you have a brain scan after." He couldn't wait to see what he learned from this, saying, "We use these extreme performers, these optimal athletes, and then we try to extract principles we can apply to the average person. It's absolutely cutting edge."

While Walshe and Naschak were planning Acheron, they found themselves a motto: "HFU," as in, "Harden the Fuck Up." But they also kept something else in mind: "Anybody can come in and kick the shit out of people. We wanted to make it thoughtful in design."

And, of course, Naschak adds, "The athletes had to get back to work afterward, so we couldn't destroy them. We wanted to press a limit, but we didn't want to keep them from working when they got back home."

The plan was for Walshe to escort the guys to Chile, where they would then venture into the wilderness with Naschak, Sanders, and a Patagonia guide.

I built the following story from interviews with Walshe and Naschak, as well as footage from the excursion, which was filmed.

It began with a midnight wake-up call that roused the men from their beds at a small Patagonia hotel. They would never know such comfort again for nearly two weeks.

In the hotel courtyard, Navy SEAL Steve Sanders showed them how to organize their hiking packs. In those packs went socks, a long-sleeve zip-neck top, a sleeping bag, ski poles, and, among many other items, crampons—spikes to strap to the bottoms of their boots in order to hike and climb on ice. Fifty pounds total.

They loaded into a van and rode three hours through dark countryside. Between the bumpy road and the anticipation, none of them slept.

At about 3:15 A.M., they unloaded beside a lake, in the Aysén Region of southern Chile, on a remote land known as the Northern Patagonian Ice Field. A fairly safe area, there was minimal wildlife, even less crime, and little risk of disease, while still being close *enough* to civilization if they needed help. It was wild land, though, broken up by steep mountains, and home to unpredictable, sometimes dangerous weather.

Wearing headlamps for light, the team boarded a twenty-one-foot fiberglass fishing boat. As they crossed Lago Bertrand, the moon showed them what lay ahead: glaciers, mountains capped by snow, the universe. They could see vast stretches of space and millions of stars.

Following Naschak, the group hiked through woods and across rugged dirt-and-rock terrain for three hours, their headlamps the only reliable light. The sun didn't break over the mountains until they'd reached a river, and their next task.

At the river, they strapped on life preservers and climbed into kayaks. Their guide, Jonathan Leidich—looking like a nineties-era Woody Harrelson in a gray Patagonia beanie—warned them: "The lake's really cold. It's only four degrees Celsius. It's only been water—like, liquid—for less than a day. It was ice last night. So the idea of the day is, don't go into the water."

They paddled seven miles down the river in their kayaks and landed on a grassy shore in the middle of a sprawling valley. Time for another hike—a much longer one, Naschak said, following the valley directly west, aiming for an ice cap called Shark's Fin. As they began the hike, Naschak said, "This is the first of one million, eight hundred fifty-seven thousand, three hundred and forty-two steps you're going to take until you leave Chile. So, enjoy."

If you were one of the guys and were just told you'd be taking nearly two million steps over the next ten days while carrying fifty pounds of hard-core survival gear, you'd probably want to know all you could about this guy Naschak. Sure, he looks the part and could probably even pass for an action-movie star, with his strong jaw and youthful appearance. But who is he, really? Why did Andy Walshe send you out into the wilderness with him?

First off, it's *Master Chief* Pete Naschak. He became a Navy SEAL in 1989, two years out of high school. He did that for twenty-one years, and on his final tour, he was the command master chief of SEAL Team Five. When he retired, he got his master's degree in global leadership and started his own company, providing consulting on teamwork, leadership, and the like, to companies such as Red Bull and Nike.

There are lots of ex-military types starting up "leadership" and "team-building" camps and seminars and consulting with companies and that sort of thing. They bother Naschak.

Not that you'd know it from talking to him. He's nice like that. Doesn't want to say anything negative about anyone. But he doesn't do the whole boot-camp-drill-sergeant, macho-man thing. He speaks with this calm, quiet voice that hums with authority. When he says something, you trust him. And he wants to make sure people understand that much of that military leadership consultation isn't based in science. It's a fun time, sure, but maybe not as helpful as it might seem. He says, "They'll go out and teach you how to do close-quarters combat, they'll take you out and do fake battles and plan missions and attack a target, and do all this stuff, and they'll do basic underwater demolition SEAL training, and other basic SEAL training they'll go through with you—and they'll go, 'You're just like us!' You're out there running around, getting yelled at, sprayed with water, and all that stuff. And that's all cool. But [it's] been done for a reason [in the military], and that's to develop a combatant. It's cool, and it's experience, but it won't translate as much, and as well, as doing it in a different format."

Naschak takes a pragmatic approach to his training, which is one reason he took the athletes to the Patagonian wilderness and not to boot camp. "They don't need to be trained to be combatants," he says. "I like to take some of those lessons that we learned, and maybe even some of the methodology, but do them in a different way, in a different environment that makes sense."

For Acheron in particular, part of Naschak's focus was disrupting these elite athletes' highly regimented lives. "Acheron is about a transformational experience," he says. "Even if they're very physical, let's get them to a point where they break down and fall apart. Athletes can be very controlling—they know what they need to do, they know how long they have to compete, they know how hard they have to compete. They've trained for it. They really know how to compete in that world and control it. So Acheron is about taking people completely out of their comfort zone of control, and then breaking them down. Not necessarily in the military sense, but getting them to the point where they don't try to game the system anymore."

And not only did Naschak want to keep them from gaming the system, he wanted to keep them immersed in what they were doing, too. To that end, no iPods, iPhones, or any such technology was allowed. "Forcing them to own their own thoughts," he says.

Naturally, Naschak draws from his own experience, and not just from when he was in the military. He says that his mother, an immigrant who fled to America from Germany during World War II, would take him and his siblings on long hikes as children.

"Up in the mountains," he says, "and basically push us to where we were crying, as little knuckleheads."

What he's learned from both that and the military is how capable we are of letting things go. "A big piece of handling combat, handling the military, is dump the small things," he says. "Don't worry about them. Control what's important. Control what you can control. And just adjust, and have the confidence to know that you *can* adjust, and make it happen."

They hiked all that first day, trekking over treacherous ground, often single file, dozens if not hundreds of feet up the side of a cliff, along ridges barely wide enough for their feet. After fourteen miles, deep in a forest, they finally made camp.

They were up before dawn on day two, and they hiked some more. By the afternoon, they were out of the woods and off solid ground, using the crampons to hike on ice. They had to jump across deep, deadly crevasses, some of them hundreds of feet deep, all of them sharp and black. To cross, they had to do what Leidich called "the most dangerous thing": use light steps and catapult themselves over using their hiking poles, taking care not to get their spikes stuck before the jump so they didn't go in headfirst. "Because," Leidich said, "you will die."

These were a bunch of individual athletes, but here they became a team, helping each other up steep hills and down sharp declines and across the occasional tricky crevasse.

They went ten miles. Along the way, surfer Ian Walsh's knee gave out. He'd hurt it months earlier, recovered enough for a doctor to clear him, but somewhere in all the hiking he had tweaked it again. By nightfall, as they make camp, he couldn't bend it.

The next morning, they were up at 3:30 A.M. They kayaked seven miles downriver, then hiked through more forest. Ian's knee required constant wrapping and bracing, and he said it felt like someone kept stabbing it. By midafternoon, they'd hiked twelve miles, and Ian couldn't bear it anymore. "My knee stopped working," he said.

They hiked to a valley, where a helicopter picked Ian up. One man down and out.

They made camp in a wooded area, and began day four like the others, before sunrise. The goal for the day was to summit Shark's Fin's peak. "We're all somehow breaking little by little," kayaker Rafa Ortiz said. "Usually when I get in a river in my kayak, you have a goal. You have something that you're reaching. And that's in the back of your mind the whole time. Here, you don't know when you're going to stop. You don't plan, you just live."

They hiked until their trail ran them into a lake, where they pulled inflatable kayaks from their packs, deployed, and paddled across. The lake had icebergs in it. On the other side, they docked on the shore of the Colonia Glacier.

Naschak reminded them, "These are parts no one has been before."

They strapped into the crampons again and hiked eight miles across the glacier. At one point they climbed straight up walls of ice, using nothing but their crampons and ice picks. "Completely at the mercy of the terrain," said Steve Sanders.

Rafa's knee started aching along the way, only growing worse with time.

They reached Shark's Fin's base around 5 P.M. Rafa was in such pain he could only lie flat on the ground. Another man down— but not out, at least not yet. Leidich stayed behind with him while Naschak, Kai Lenny, Matt Poole, and Sanders pushed up the mountain.

They went two thousand feet up. There was no trail, since nobody had ever climbed it before. "Damn near vertical shrubbery," is how Matt Poole described it. "A nightmare. A jungle."

After twenty-one hours of hiking, kayaking, and climbing over a five-thousand-foot increase in elevation—"twenty-one hours of fun," Naschak called it—they found a flat spot to make camp. Flurries began to fall.

Day five started early, too, with 4,500 more feet of elevation to cover before reaching the summit. But the flurries became all-out snowfall, and with no trail and snow up to their knees, they had to take slow, careful steps. Between the thick shrubbery and the relentless snow, the going went from tough to literally impossible as the path became too dangerous.

They weren't going to make it. Naschak turned the group around and they returned to base camp.

The wake-up call for day six was 5 A.M. Lenny said, "I love that nowadays that sounds so late."

They inflated their rafts and paddled for half the morning until the river reached an impasse. They packed up the rafts and climbed until they reached level ground, and then they hiked all day across what looked like nothing but rocks. Then they pulled the rafts back out of their packs and inflated them again and paddled some more, then they docked again, packed up the rafts again, and loaded themselves into one big raft and took on some white water for a couple hours.

The day ended with their meeting Andy Walshe at a farm. They'd put in a total of four miles hiking and seven miles paddling, covering a grand total of ninety miles in six days. They feasted—lamb, potatoes, salad, wine—and reflected. All of them said they'd had tremendous highs, yes, but that they were also all breaking.

Naschak told them, "I get asked all the time . . . how do our guys work in such close, tight units? It's like we *know* each other. We think alike. And we perform at high levels—we make these big decisions in life-and-death arenas. This is exactly how we do it. It's because we go through training, we go through periods like this . . . Doing stuff for *fun,* which pushes us, and breaks us down. And we suffer. And we laugh. And we deal with it all, together."

For day seven, they paddled for seven hours to cover twenty-five miles of river, including a great deal of white water.

Day eight began at 4 A.M., hiking through darkness using head-lamps, their sights set on another mountain. The mountain didn't have a name, so they named it Cana Brava. Elevation 6,500 feet. As the sun rose, the path looked more promising than the path at Shark's Fin had, no shrubbery, little snowfall, mostly rocks. As the hours went by, all hiking boots and poles and exhaustion, Kai Lenny said, "Project Acheron—all of a sudden that name made a lot more sense. To get where I wanna go, I'm going to have to push myself. I'm going to have to hurt to get there."

In the early afternoon, after fourteen straight hours of hiking, they reached the summit. Naschak told them, "This is un-touched."

When they returned to camp beside the river late that night, Poole, Ortiz, and Lenny decided to celebrate by stripping to their underwear and diving in the four-degree Celsius water.

Up at dawn once again for day nine, they were sore from climbing Cana Brava. Once they'd packed and were ready to re-board the raft, Naschak pulled the group together. "Had a badass day yesterday," he said. "Now we've got ourselves a paddle." He pointed across the river. To the other shore. "It's really just right over to there. And then we're done. That's the day. And then that's it. We start heading back home. You guys did it."

Back at UCSD, the guys were tested same as before. Their EEG scans showed more stable brain-wave activity. More alpha, less beta. Their brains were more resilient to stress, more stable with their emotions, and better at making hard decisions under stress. Also, the fMRI scans showed real changes to their brain structure, particularly in Migsby, who is, you probably remember by now, the key component of the brain's fear system. Under stressful conditions, far less blood got to Migsby, meaning that Migsby had become much calmer than before Acheron.

In other words, Acheron physically altered how their brains processed fear.

In the past, this might have been seen as just some sort of spirit quest, and we might think, "Oh, good for them."

But those test results—that was spirituality quantified.

All of that is fine and good, but for their purposes, the expedition wouldn't matter if it didn't translate to their performance.

But it did.

Matt Poole told Naschak he realized that he'd lost his reason for being in his sport. "He had gotten into racing for sponsors, and not for himself," Naschak says. "And he said the trip changed him. Flipped the switch. He came back stronger, with a whole different shift in mind-set—he wasn't in awe of the number one guy anymore. He didn't look *up* to the stars anymore. He acted like he was their peer."

Kai Lenny's transformation was maybe even more profound. He'd gone into this a boy, but he wasn't a boy afterward. Kai's father told Naschak, "You took my son away, and you gave me back a different person. He's a man now."

In the year after Acheron, Lenny won two stand-up paddleboarding world titles, placed second in the world in kite surfing, and caught the biggest barrels and waves of his life.

Chapter 18

Psychedelica

Going into 2010, Kyle Kingsbury's career as a six-foot-four, 205-pound light heavyweight fighter in the UFC hadn't been as good as some others, but it was as good as he could have hoped for when he started fighting as a pro just four years earlier, which happened basically by accident.

He'd been a football player. Defensive lineman, team captain at Monta Vista High School in Cupertino, twice all-league, second-team All Central Coast Section his senior year, followed by a couple years at Arizona State, where he wasn't a star but still got his minutes, including during ASU's 2004 Sun Bowl championship.

After college, he wanted to stay in shape, but he was easily bored by lifting weights and running. "I needed some kind of physical interaction," he says.

He started martial arts training, with no plans to fight, but the owner of his gym ran a local fight promotion, told Kingsbury he had real potential, and talked him into trying a fight. "Just do it once," the guy said. "If you like it, you can keep doing it. If you don't like it, you don't have to do it ever again."

Kingsbury was no stranger to fighting. He had a temper. He tells me, "I wouldn't say I was an angry person. I was a happy person. But, in an instant, I could be at this high level of anger. I wouldn't call it a blind rage, but certainly not a healthy level of anger."

One of the best ways he found to release that anger as a kid was by fighting. As it turned out, that anger was helpful in the cage. He had, in his words, "a burning desire to hurt someone," and hurt people he did. He won his first fight in June 2006 by knockout—in nineteen seconds. "If you ever knock somebody out," he says, "it's the equivalent of hitting a home run, times a thousand. It's the most addictive feeling on earth."

Kingsbury, who has done his share of weed, ecstasy, mushrooms, and more, adds, "There's no drug like it."

A mere three weeks later, he fought his second pro fight—and knocked out his opponent in twenty-nine seconds.

He fought three more times by the end of the year, winning all but one by knockout or submission in under two minutes. He didn't lose until three fights later, in September 2007.

After that, he moved from Phoenix to San Jose, California, to prepare for the UFC by training at the American Kickboxing Academy, home of UFC greats Frank Shamrock and Cain Velasquez, the latter of whom, in addition to being a two-time UFC heavyweight champion, had gone to Arizona State with Kingsbury.

Kingsbury spent about a year training at AKA, where he made much-needed improvements, before making his run at the UFC with a couple months in Vegas as part of the cast for *The Ultimate Fighter,* the UFC reality show on Spike TV. Sixteen fighters are split into two teams and compete. Kingsbury lost by decision in the season finale.

In his first UFC fight at UFC 104 in October 2009 in Los Angeles, he won by split decision. He'd fought well, but, he says, "There was still something missing—I wasn't good at clearing my mind."

No matter what, it seemed like Kingsbury's anger kept burning hot, and might have even been getting worse. Fire in the belly can be good, but wildfire in the heart can burn everything down. He'd tried meditation, visualization, and some other methods of claiming control of his mind, but he could not calm down, especially going into a fight. At prefight weigh-ins, in particular, he was a mess, anger frequently giving way to panic attacks. He worked with multiple sports psychologists and therapists, talking through the anger and anxiety. Best they could figure, the roots went back to his childhood.

Kingsbury had grown up watching his parents fight all the time. They were married fourteen years, and, Kingsbury says, "For the majority of the time, they were fighting, or yelling at each other. There were very few good memories of all of us getting along at the same time. And it just blew my mind that they lived that way for that long."

Kingsbury is quick to add, "I know many, many people have it worse than I did. I'm not saying I had it *that* bad. But at the same time, kids don't need to see that shit. And it certainly affected me."

Even finding a root for his anger, however, didn't make the anger go away. No matter his work with therapists, Kingsbury says, "It never got ironed out. It didn't matter how much we talked about it, or used different techniques. None of that ever subsided."

Before every fight camp—the eight weeks before the fight— Kingsbury and his boxing coach, a man of Mexican and Native

American descent, went to a Native American reservation to do a traditional *temazcal*. Basically, it's a sweat lodge. Their goal, Kingsbury says, was always pretty much the same: clear the mind, set a course of action, dial in the purpose of the next two months. (They'd also return after each fight "for reflection and healing.")

That's what they did in 2010 in the run-up to Kingsbury's September fight against Jared Hamman. This time, Kingsbury asked the guide, "When are we going to do this the traditional way—when are we going to add in the plant medicine?"

The guide smiled a big smile and said he'd been waiting for Kyle to ask.

By "plant medicine," Kingsbury meant psilocybin mushrooms.

He was familiar with them. He'd done them plenty of times before, once even having a breakthrough experience that felt transcendent while in the desert of Sedona, Arizona. "But that was just by chance," he says.

His guide at the reservation, he says, "showed it to me a different way."

The guide blessed the mushrooms, and, with Kyle, asked for their guidance. Kingsbury says, "This isn't just some street drug you take for a good time. You have an intention, and you have a reason for going, a reason for doing this." That would become much more important years later.

Meanwhile, Kingsbury went on to win his fight that September by unanimous decision. He used mushrooms with his *temazcal* every time after that—and, whether a credit to the psychedelic addition to his training or not, over the next year, he won two more fights, one by knockout and the other by unanimous decision.

He had himself a winning streak, just the thing an elite UFC fighter needs.

Problem was, though the mushrooms helped him in some ways, even they could not eliminate his anger and fear. If anything, they only kept getting worse, because with every fight, he became more scared of losing. He says, "You have to have a healthy fear, and respect for your opponent. If you go in there thinking, *I'm gonna just walk through this guy,* nine times out of ten, you're gonna get your ass kicked, even if you're better than him. So there's a level of respect and fear that must come with any engagement in battle. But, that said, I had more than that. I had a greater fear. I had a greater fear of the consequences of loss."

One of his biggest worries was money. He says, "In the UFC, they double your win, so if I made ten grand to show up, and then an additional ten grand to win, that's not a lot of money if you lose, and even if I win, it's barely enough to stay afloat. And that might be the only fight I have that year. Well, twenty grand after you pay the IRS, and your coaches, ain't shit. It's poverty level wherever you live, and in the Bay Area, it's damn sure poverty level. So there's the pressure there, to succeed, to build a win streak."

And he was succeeding. That's the thing. He won two Fight of the Night bonuses, in fact, including one for his knockout, which took just twenty-one seconds. (Knees to the body and punches.) He was being considered as a potential light heavyweight championship contender.

Yet, in his mind, "The pressure kept building."

And then he lost.

And lost and lost.

In less than a year, he lost one fight by unanimous decision, another by submission, and worst of all, in September 2012, he lost by technical knockout. He nearly submitted rookie fighter Jimi Manuwa in seconds, dodging a wild left hook and decking Jimi with a punch of his own, climbing on, and almost choking him out. They spent two full minutes grappling before Manuwa got free. Then Manuwa unloaded on Kyle, putting him on his back multiple times, one powerful punch and kick after another, nearly knocking him out. "He ate so many shots that would have knocked out many of the 205-pounders out there," one of the broadcasters said.

Somehow, despite his left eye swelling shut, Kingsbury stayed in it, and pounded Manuwa during an electric second round. The round ended with Kingsbury on top of Manuwa, giving him one elbow after another. But then when he rose grinning from the mat, the crowd gasped in shock, and the ring doctor rushed to his corner to examine him: his left eye was swollen beyond closed, a little purple balloon. The doctor and referee agreed that if Kingsbury couldn't see, then he couldn't keep fighting. He tried to open the eye—and the crowd shrieked more—but he couldn't see.

The ref raised his arms and waved them.

The fight was over.

At the hospital, Kyle learned that he'd suffered two orbital bone fractures and that he had torn his left labrum. Less than two weeks after the fight, he told a reporter that he was pretty sure he would never fight again.

Sometime—he's not exactly sure when—between the Manuwa loss and the end of 2012, Kyle was talking to a buddy, Brandon Rhinehart, who was on a trip to Peru, "doing some soul-searching." Rhinehart called when he arrived and said that he was there for a week, and he could either do a five-day trek of Machu Picchu—the renowned fifteenth-century Incan citadel high in the Andes Mountains above the Urubamba River valley—or, he said, "I can do this stuff called ayahuasca."

Kingsbury said, "Well, fucking hike Machu Picchu. What are you thinking, dude? I've never heard of this ayahuasca stuff."

"Look it up," Rhinehart said. "It's supposed to be a pretty potent psychedelic."

"You can do psychedelics anywhere," Kingsbury said. "Go hike Machu Picchu."

So Rhinehart did. But meanwhile, Kingsbury got curious and googled ayahuasca. And he said, *Wait a minute.* The first thing he saw: *apex of teacher plants.*

"This is the top of the heap," he says now. "This is the most powerful, most potent, most transcendent thing you can do."

Ayahuasca is a brew made, in fact, out of two different plants, and is deeply significant to the indigenous Amazonian tribes. Those who have drunk it consider it everything from medicine to a key to a portal into the spiritual dimension. (It's also illegal in the United States.) In the Amazon, shamans figured out how to make it some unknown many years ago, using a combination of one plant's leaf and another plant's vine. Making the brew takes about ten hours, and it has to be cooked in big, cast-iron pots. The payoff: ayahuasca delivers the most powerful psychedelic drug known to man, Dimethyltryptamine, commonly known as DMT.

The human body naturally produces DMT within itself; the brew just gives you a whole lot more of it.

That ayahuasca exists at all is some kind of miracle. The leaf and vine come from two very different plants that don't grow anywhere near each other in the Amazonian jungles. The shamans say the plants taught them how to make it—and they get offended when people call it a drug. To them, it is sacred medicine.

Kingsbury called his coach and said, "Hey, we gotta go to Peru. I don't speak very good Spanish, and this is something I really want to try."

His coach said, "We'll bring Peru to us."

They found some traveling shamans who met them at their Native American reservation. For two weeks prior to the ayahuasca date, Kingsbury was told to follow a strict *dieto,* eating light, clean, and organic. No junk food, all that. "Strictly forbidden," he says.

Kingsbury and his coach arrived the night before the ayahuasca ceremony and did the standard *temazcal,* without adding any psychedelics. Then he slept.

Although most ayahuasca ceremonies take place at night, Kingsbury's began the next morning. He had fasted for nearly twenty-four hours by that point. Some shamans begin the ceremony with elaborate chanting and singing. Kingsbury's was more simple. He and his coach arrived, they got situated—there were several other people there for the ceremony—and then they all took a Solo cup's worth of ayahuasca.

It was thick and gritty, almost sludge, tasting of earth and fire. Kingsbury washed his down with a little water.

Then he sat and waited.

Nothing happened the first hour. A little sweat, nothing more.

He was offered a second cup. He took it. Then he lay down.

Moments later, a noise began to escalate rapidly until Kingsbury felt like he was in a war zone, surrounded by roars and screaming.

He remembered something he was told before. *Respect the Noble Silence.* Don't look around. Don't eavesdrop if you can help it. Let other people have their experience to themselves, and have your own experience. Because, he was told, most people have visceral reactions to ayahuasca. They weep, laugh, scream.

Kingsbury kept his eyes closed, and when he couldn't, he looked down. The sounds, though, were horrible. "Like people dying," he said. And he couldn't help but look.

The others were "puking horribly."

This, too, is a key component of the ayahuasca experience. The purge. *La purga.* You vomit. You have diarrhea. You purge.

Everyone was given a bucket, and most people were using

theirs now, but Kingsbury felt like his would remain clean. And he began to judge.

Nobody around him was as healthy as he was. As fit as he was. None of them respected their bodies like he did. None of them ate properly. He remembered them, the night before, breaking the fast, eating, he says, "potato chips and shit, like they were at a campsite." So he thought, *Well, there it is. Of course they're going to turn themselves inside out. They weren't paying attention to the diet. They're not healthy individuals.*

And then Kingsbury recognized that old, familiar anger. That hot fire. His thoughts grew harsher and darker. He thought about not only the unhealthy people with him, but also, he says, "all these fat people who have disgusted me in my life." He thought about fat people he'd seen drive a motorized cart into a McDonald's. He would glare at them, burning inside with rage. How could someone *destroy* themselves that way?

He caught himself. He thought, *Why the fuck would anyone TAKE this stuff? All I feel is this anger. All I feel—oh shit . . .*

He lurched up and grabbed his bucket, and he puked harder than he'd ever puked in his life.

La purga.

As he purged, he realized that his anger was leaving him with every retch.

When the puking stopped, he felt something he'd never felt before. He felt lighter, and he felt compassion, a warmth in his heart. "My whole life," he says, "I've been an athlete. I learned at a very young age that what you put in your body can help you perform better. And so I saw this correlation between food, and feeling good, that most people don't see. And I had this compassion for people who never knew it that way. They never understood it. Maybe every time their parents got in a fight, their dad would take them to McDonald's for an ice cream cone, and say, 'Hey, don't worry about it, kiddo. Here you go.' Maybe there was some other food attachment that led to eating the wrong foods in times of stress. Whatever the case may be, maybe they just ate like crap their whole life because they don't know any better. That, really, was a huge release for me. I didn't even know how deep that had gone, this anger toward people that don't take care of themselves. But as that left me, I could see it for what it was. And I knew it wasn't healthy—it was this nasty emotion I had inside, and I was able to release it."

He set the bucket down and started sweating profusely, then he collapsed and starting shaking.

One of the guides said, "Should we check him? Is he okay?"

"No," his coach said. "Leave him alone. He's gotta work through it."

At that, Kingsbury stopped shaking, but he sweated even more. He rubbed at his eyes to get the sweat out of them—and in that moment he felt greater euphoria than he'd ever felt. "Euphoria," he says, "times a thousand. I took ecstasy plenty of times back in the day. This was way, way, *wayyy* more so. I was almost in disbelief of how good it felt. I've taken things in the past for the physical pleasure of it, and knowing full well it's just for the physical pleasure of it, but that's not why I was here. I was here to learn. I was here to grow. So I thought of my first intention, and I thought of myself as this fighter."

And, he says, "That's when everything broke down."

It was almost like *Fight Club*, the thoughts that started going through his head. "You're not your car. You're not your clothes. You're not the books you read. You're not the house you own. You're none of these things." He says, "[My mind] really just disassembled everything I thought of myself, in terms of my identity. I'm not my name. I'm not Kyle Kingsbury. This is just something I've been given in this world, for people to call me, and understand. There was zero attachment to anything at that point. And it just blew my mind."

As he lay there, his eyes closed, feeling attached to nothing and euphoric about it, he hadn't begun hallucinating yet—except for one thing that, for some reason, most people who drink ayahuasca or smoke DMT see: a kaleidoscope of polygons and other shapes, mixed with bright orange, red, and yellow backgrounds. The shamans call it *"the Sacred Geometry."*

Kingsbury says, "I was looking at this like, *Holy shit, I've never seen anything so magnificent in my life!* But again, I was reminded, *Okay, I'm not here just to look at this cool stuff."*

He was there to sort out his feelings about fighting—and then he found peace about it almost instantly, in just over an hour. Knowing full well he had a good six, seven hours of ayahuasca high to go, he wasn't sure what to do next. He remembered one of the guides saying, "If you reach your intention, and you feel like you got everything you want from it, you can think of loved ones, and think of people close to you, and you'll gain a new perspective."

Natasha. His girlfriend. He thought of her. And instantly, he slipped into a vision in which he *was* her, looking up at him—he saw himself, his own face and long hair and beard. He looked down, and he *was* Natasha. He had her hair, her body. And Natasha was screaming at Kyle. He relived every argument they ever had. "And everything I was saying, as Natasha," Kingsbury says now, "was in a way that Kyle would understand it."

After he pulled out of the vision sometime later, he says, "It changed me forever. I realized that her intention, in every argument, was love. It wasn't about, you know, making me feel like shit for going out and drinking the night before. It wasn't about me not wanting to see my friends, or whatever the case may be, for the argument's sake. I understood that it was love, and that really changed my relationship with her. And I cried like a little kid."

He laughs. "I couldn't even tell you this story for about two weeks after the fact. That's how lasting and deep this was for me. And when I told Natasha—same deal. I broke down."

And he wasn't done yet.

Next he thought of his mom. "Being a thirty-however-old guy, everyone doesn't see eye to eye with their mom," he says. "I don't need to give you a background story on that."

But when he thought of her, same as he'd become Natasha, now he became Mom, and he was pregnant with baby Kyle. He says, "I was her with her first child inside her. I wasn't Kyle inside my mom. I *was* my mom, as a brand-new parent-to-be, with this child growing inside me."

In a time lapse, he watched his belly grow bigger. And he saw his father. "Rick would come over and kiss the belly," he says, "and kiss me, and encourage me, as my mom. And I felt the nervousness of wanting to do right. Of wanting to be the best parent I could be. I felt the anxiety of being a new parent. And I felt this genuine, unconditional love through my body, just wash over me like a warm blanket, from my father and my mother, with Kyle growing inside."

Then he pulled out of the vision. He didn't have children, but at that moment he understood what parents mean when they say, "You won't know what it's like until you have kids of your own."

He lay there looking up at the sky. Trees stretched across the horizon. And from the tops of the trees, he saw ripples drifting through the air from tree to tree, like the sky was water. "Like they were communicating with each other," he says.

That first trip lasted from about 10 A.M. until about 6 P.M.

Kingsbury did ayahuasca a few more times over the next two years. Somewhere along the way, his anger, his desire to hurt somebody, dissolved. He's not sure which ceremony did it. Probably the combination of all of them, he says. But if it was any single one of them, he says, it was his fourth one, in early 2013, when he focused not on anger, but on fear.

Once again, Kyle needed two cups to get going, and after he threw up a bunch, he was so exhausted that he dropped his face nearly into his bucket full of puke. Then, he says, "I cried like I hadn't cried in years. I mean, even the other ayahuasca ceremonies didn't compare to this level of crying. It was opening the floodgates. And I just went with it. This is something, I figured, I haven't done in a while, and I need to get this out, and it's okay to cry."

It went on so long it became alarming. *Why can't I stop crying? Why am I STILL crying?*

Then Kyle's first vision started. He was seven years old, in his childhood bedroom, sitting on his bunk bed, the door closed. His parents were screaming at each other in the living room. Old terror flashed alive in him, and then anger rose, too, as though to protect him from the fear. He kept crying, and his mind reverted to the way he thought when he was that little. *Why do they fight so much?*

And then he saw *their* fear. "It showed me their fears as parents," he says. "Their fears of money, of being able to pay rent, to put food on the table. How much they're working. Feeling underappreciated. Fearing they're underappreciated by their partner. All this awful stuff—it stemmed from fear. And instead of having anger toward them—like, *Look what you did!*—or any of that stuff, it was just this deep compassion for them. Like, *holy shit*, I couldn't believe they had lived that way."

That gave rise to another question in Kingsbury's mind: *What fear do I live with?*

"And right then," he says, "it showed me the fear I have every time I get in the cage."

The fears of pressure, of money—or lack thereof—and the

fears of losing. He saw all the many times he had been too afraid. And then he saw . . . Anderson Silva, the middleweight legend who holds the longest title streak in UFC history of 2,457 days, sixteen straight wins, and ten title defenses. *Why am I seeing Anderson Silva?* he thought. Then Kyle realized—and this sums up why his story resonates so deeply with stories like my own—that, "What makes [Silva] great, what makes him one of the best ever, is that, even though he gets nervous, he doesn't fear any more than is necessary. His deepest belief is a belief in himself. Even if [his opponent is] better than him in any department of the fight game, he believes in himself, and he believes he's gonna win. That really showed me what unnecessary fears I had—and what unnecessary fears I had seen growing up, and how they impacted my life, and how much pain there was because of that. But as I worked through that pain, maybe that was the pain that I needed, to want to destroy someone in front of me."

In 2014, Kingsbury took his first fight in two years, right in his hometown of San Jose. (The UFC higher-ups were happy to have him fighting again, but they asked him to please not, you know, talk about all that ayahuasca stuff.)

He wanted to fight again because he wanted to see how real this change was in the one world he knew would test him. He wanted to know if he had really changed.

No competitor worth a damn is okay with losing. But could he be at peace in the face of loss?

So, in so many ways, taking another fight was really less about winning the fight against the other guy and more about winning the fight against himself.

During every training camp of his life, he was brutally hard on himself. If he had a day he didn't feel he had performed as well in his training, or his sparring, or his wrestling, or whatever else, he beat himself up about it well into the night and even the next day. *I NEED to be BETTER* echoed around him like a drill sergeant's mantra. "Overboard," he says. That old anger, he directed at himself as much as anyone else. "But I didn't have that critique of myself leading up to this fight," he says. "It just wasn't there."

Training went well. So did the prefight weigh-ins: for the first and only weigh-in of his career he didn't have a panic attack.

And then came the fight itself.

To quote MMAJunkie.com: "He lost about as badly as you can lose and still go the distance."

His fourth straight loss. In front of thousands of people. Worse, in his hometown. And yet Kingsbury said after the fight, "I definitely got what I was looking for."

And, he said, "I was at peace the entire time."

He got his ass kicked, sure, but only by the other guy that kept hitting him. Against the guy he really went in there to fight, that old angry fire monster in his heart, Kingsbury prevailed.

As of this writing, in August 2016, Kingsbury has not fought again and has no plans to. He has, however, used ayahuasca more than a dozen times. Many of those have involved actually going to the source, to Peru and the Amazon, taking dingy canoes down rivers full of monsters and sleeping in huts surrounded by jungles full of jaguars and all manner of other wild beasts. "Each trip," he says, "is completely unique."

He still gets angry. But it's normal anger. The anger he felt before, by comparison, was like a wildfire he has now put out. "There are still things I get passionate about, politically and things like that, but at the same time, that pales in comparison to where I was before. So in terms of quality of life, that's been greatly enhanced."

This is getting into some really weird territory. I know that, so I want to point out that Kingsbury, who talked with me for a couple of hours about his experiences, came off as remarkably grounded. He openly admits how weird it all seems, and he's well aware of the general public's perception of psychedelics.

I also want to acknowledge the obvious: it seems like ayahuasca might have actually hurt Kingsbury as a fighter. In fact, MMA-Junkie.com's short piece about his experience a couple of years ago ran with that very headline: "How Kyle Kingsbury Used Ayahuasca to Become a Happier Person and a Worse Fighter." The piece infuriated Kingsbury at first—ironic, right?—until he realized it might be true. But he points out that his goal in using ayahuasca wasn't to get better at fighting other people, but at managing the fight within himself. So in a way, he actually did get better as a fighter.

The point is, he got what he needed.

And while ayahuasca might not have given Kingsbury the win against his opponent, it has been given credit for helping one of his UFC cohorts to do just that.

In May 2012, Dan Hardy knocked out Duane Ludwig in the first round of his undercard match at UFC 146 at the MGM Grand, then he went for a trip. He left Vegas and spent two weeks in a small wooden hut in the jungles of Peru, where, among other things, he did ayahuasca three times.

Months later, Hardy was still struggling to put the experience into words. He had several visions—at one point breathing fire—and he met a wolf that he could touch. He has a hard time describing it, but he it changed him. A onetime CWFC welterweight champion and near UFC welterweight and light welterweight champion—losing a title fight to legend Georges St.-Pierre—Hardy credited ayahuasca with helping him refocus.

Later that year, in September, he fought and defeated Amir Sadollah by unanimous decision.

Kingsbury knows a *lot* of other athletes, some of them better than he ever was, doing the exact same thing as he did. Many of them have their own unique experience, though all follow a more or less similar emotional and spiritual track. There are several other UFC fighters who are using ayahuasca, and he's talked with many athletes in other sports—including some NFL players, among others—who are exploring it, too.

These other athletes, whether in UFC or the NFL or the NBA or elsewhere, won't go public as of this writing in fall 2016. They are still competing, some of them at the apex of their field, and thus have way more to lose. Mainstream culture—not to mention their teams and bosses—probably wouldn't respond all that well to hearing about their athletes taking trips to Peru and Native American reservations to ingest a psychedelic brew that makes them hallucinate for hours on end.

That's why I think it's also important to draw attention to some fascinating studies being conducted by the scientific and medical communities on psychedelics such as ayahuasca.

The writer Kira Salak recently wrote a story for *National Geographic* that described how she was cured of lifelong depression after drinking ayahuasca. Many others have shared how it helped treat their depression, too, as well as anxiety, OCD, fibromyalgia, and PTSD. An organization known as MAPS (Multidisciplinary Association for Psychedelic Studies) has been conducting numerous studies on several drugs for treating PTSD, such as ecstasy, LSD, and ayahuasca. Biomedical researchers are checking it out. And while the results are skimpy, they are promising: several military veterans suffering from PTSD have felt a dramatic sense of peace after an ayahuasca experience, overcoming suicidal urges, anger, rage, and depression. One soldier described it to CNN as a "psychedelic baptism."

Psychiatrist Brian Anderson from the University of California–San Francisco recently told *Scientific American*, "The relationship between ayahuasca's psychedelic effects and its therapeutic effects needs to be empirically studied."

According to *Scientific American,* "It is biochemically plausible that ayahuasca could treat depression." The DMT in ayahuasca binds to your brain's serotonin receptors, which help you feel pleasure, and other chemicals in ayahuasca—harmine, tetrahydroharmine, and harmaline—inhibit the enzyme *monoamine oxidase A,* which prevents the breakdown of serotonin and other neurotransmitters.

On the Tim Ferriss Show, a podcast by the bestselling author and investor, a hospice doctor, BJ Miller, told Ferriss that he knew a former colleague who left hospice care to do illegal work with such drugs. He said that the woman did this because the experience of one's impending death is profound and full of revelations, and she wanted to find a way to give it to people before they actually died so they could live better lives. And, he said, she's told him that now she watches people die every weekend, and then come back to life.

Kingsbury says he's heard plenty of skepticism and even cynicism regarding the use of ayahuasca. In a way, he gets it. "Ten years ago," he says, "people would've told you if you took psilocybin mushrooms, 'It's gonna fry your brain.' My uncle told me that when I was a kid! But now at Johns Hopkins University, there are studies showing that not only does it not fry the brain, it *heals* the brain. It heals damaged tissue. It opens up blood flow and new neural networks and cross-flow between multiple parts of the brain that don't usually interact with one another, and that's what allows for the perspectives and the visuals. So the more we understand, scientifically, about these things, the more we'll come to realize these plants aren't hurting anyone. And the fact that they can expand consciousness, and awareness, and our appreciation for the world, and enhance our quality of life—that should be a pretty big priority to help move things in that direction, and help end this bullshit prohibition that we've been wasting money on for thirty years."

Kingsbury is done fighting, though. San Jose was the end of all that. He has fought that fire in his heart into submission. "That burning desire to hurt someone left me," he says. "And I can credit that to ayahuasca."

Also, remember Natasha? They're married now. And they have a child.

He's thirty-four, still young enough for a comeback (fans ask). He still trains, but it's just to stay in shape. He still loves the sport, but he's a little tired of getting punched in the face, and besides, he says, "There's more to life than fighting."

He's working as a bartender and a bouncer now, and preparing to start a new career.

He's going to be a firefighter.

Chapter 19

Deprivation

Naked in the dark and floating in space, I see, hear, and feel nothing.

I'm not *really* in space. I'm in Los Angeles, at a place called Float Lab, in Westwood, lying in a big tub full of shin-deep skin-temperature water and a thousand pounds of Epsom salt.

This is a sensory deprivation chamber, also known as a float tank. The idea is to completely remove any and all physical sensation, leaving only you and your mind.

With this, we're back to Steph Curry. He got into float tanks before the 2015 season after the Warriors' new head of physical performance and sports science, Lachlan Penfold, told the team to check it out. Curry got hooked. He openly talked with ESPN reporter Sam Alipour in 2016 about how he goes for a good float at least once a week, typically at Reboot Spa in San Francisco. Alipour said Curry's weekly floats might be one of his big secrets.

That said, Curry's far from the only athlete floating—his teammate Harrison Barnes joined him and Alipour later, and Barnes usually goes with Curry and Curry's wife, Ayesha, for their weekly floats. Beyond the NBA, athletes from football to mixed martial arts to skateboarding to golf have been connected to floating in one way or another. Ohio State football has a tank in their training facility right next to the hot tubs. Tom Brady's into floating, as is Houston Texans All-Pro defensive end J. J. Watt. The guy who owns Float Lab told me that Red Bull's athletes come in for floats all the time, as do many different pro athletes and other celebrities. He also helped build a chamber for former Bulls great Elton Brand, installing one in his home before arguably Brand's best season of his career.

What neither Curry nor any of the rest get into is how trippy a good sensory-deprived float can be, especially your first few times. For one thing, the magnesium in the salt is good for sore muscles, and spending an hour or two suspended weightless decompresses the spine and eases out tension.

Moreover, the time spent taking in literally *nothing* seems to be fantastic for your mind. Curry doesn't go too deep about it—all he's said is that he likes the chance to relax, "to get away from the demands and all the stimuli we have in the world in our lives. That was the main draw."

With nothing to do or see or feel, your mind starts showing you things that aren't physically there. Our brains naturally create narratives to make sense out of whatever we're experiencing, whether it's what's going on around us or within us.

Research has found that a sensory deprivation experience rivals that of a meditation expert reaching a peak meditative state. In many ways, the research I found echoes a lot of what NuCalm does for the mind, brain, and body. Sensory deprivation drives the brain first into alpha-brain-wave territory, but then even further, into the theta range, with EEG scans reflecting brain activity similar to what occurs when someone is asleep. A 2009 study found that just fifteen minutes of sensory deprivation is enough to make people have vivid hallucinations.

Cut off all outside sensory input and all your brain is left to work with is whatever you've got floating around inside. For some, that's frightening, at least at first, but for many—especially those who are first afraid—it can be quite healing.

Curry's go-to float spot, Reboot in San Francisco, was directly inspired by Float Lab—and the guy who created Float Lab was inspired by that potential for healing. He needed it.

Meet Crash. About five-foot-ten, short, uncombed brown hair, ragged Float Lab T-shirt, cutoff jean shorts, sandals. And sunglasses. Always sunglasses. He's passionate about Float Lab but not in the scary sort of zealot way; you can just tell how much he believes in this stuff by how meticulous he is with the details of his operation, with how cheap he prices sessions—forty dollars for two hours, an absolute steal compared to most places that charge anywhere from fifty to a hundred dollars or more for just *one* hour—and by how he rants about those other places, which he feels are ripping people off, in more ways than one.

Crash started Float Lab in 1999. Before that, he lived many lives. For work, he was an audio engineer and occasional voice actor, and he was deep into the music scene, which very much included drugs. "Narcotics, mannnn," he says. "I used to *love* to get high. And I would *get HIGH*."

He has a rich, deep voice that resonates, snappy and crisp. When he's focused, there's nobody easier to listen to. When he's not, he'll go off on long tangents full of broken sentences, like his mouth can't keep up with all his thoughts.

By the late nineties, when he was in his late thirties, Crash got tired of getting high. "It wasn't like the olden days," he says. "Back when it was, you know, a different camaraderieship with the cats that were involved in the scene. That all went away. Everybody became different. Creepy. Real creepy. Like, no honor amongst the thieves anymore, you know? I was never a rotten junkie, someone that would set you up and steal your money. Like, most of them will do that now. You don't want to fuck around with a junkie, because there's *tendencies.* And I wanted to continue to be a decent individual. I don't steal. I work."

Crash worked in Hollywood at the time, renting out sixteen rehearsal studios. "Two buildings full of fucking crazy kids," he says. "I mean, just, like, three hundred kids in there. Every door you opened up, there was another scene in there going on. Hollywood and Vine, you know? It used to be zany back then . . . I had enough and wanted to just quit."

He quit renting out the studios, then quit Los Angeles altogether, renting a ranch some ten miles south of Vegas, quitting people.

And he quit drugs, too. Well, narcotics. He still loved—still loves—some weed. But everything else, dunzo. "After twenty-five years of narcotics, just stopped," he says. He wanted a break from it all. He wanted to focus on *his* music after decades of helping other people make theirs. He had a band, and they'd had smatterings of success, and come a lucky break or two away from something that could maybe be big. He doesn't elaborate, only saying, "I'd been denied a couple of times, previously, on opportunities that almost made it my way, and then I—well, something occurred, and I was left standing there in a very unfortunate mind frame."

Out on the ranch, he built his own recording studio. "The whole fucking thing," he says. "Tape machine, analog, digital, too, and processing. It was a really great little situation."

But as he worked he was struggling with a pain, a bitterness. About every day he'd go sit in a room on a couch in front of a wall with a movie projected on it, and he'd crank up the music as loud as he could, and just sit. "I was back at the beginning again," he says. "That happened to me on different occasions, where I just destroyed things that I built. I had worked my way up time and time again and created stuff, and then fucked it up with too much fun, too much craziness, with—you know, chicks and stuff. You're out there too far. And it's hard to pull shit together when you're that far out."

The ranch had these big barrels scattered everywhere that used to—well, hold water for horses, or something, he figured. One day, he stuck his head in a barrel to sing. (It was empty.) Better for hearing how your voice sounds. Acoustics and all. Except this time, his mind went to work in there. Something about the darkness and the hearing nothing and such. When he pulled his head out, he had a thought. *I'm supposed to build these.*

"I don't even know—what *is* a deprivation chamber?" he says now, cackling at himself.

He figured the thought must've worked its way free from somewhere in his memory bank—at some point he'd seen the 1980 movie *Altered States,* the film adaptation of the Paddy Chayefsky novel that came out in 1978. It's based on the work of Dr. John C. Lilly, a well-known physician, neuroscientist, psychoanalyst, prolific writer, philosopher, inventor—and psychonaut. Among many endeavors while working with the National Institute of Mental Health, Lilly invented the sensory deprivation tank in 1954. Then came the sixties, and he experimented with LSD and the anesthetic ketamine, which he began using regularly in experiments on himself in the tank.

In *Altered States,* a doctor based on Lilly performs the same types of experiments—and eventually begins a genetic regression that turns him into a monkey.

Crash wasn't feeling the whole turn-into-a-monkey thing, but after singing in the barrel, he felt like he'd received some sort of divine message. "It was the weirdest thing *ever,*" he says. "It was just, all of a sudden, when I pulled my head out of that thing, I was a different person. One of the effects that went along with that realization was that I was no longer upset with my position in life."

Not that he had the foggiest clue how to actually build a sensory deprivation chamber. He wasn't even sure they were a real thing until he began to do some research. He found a book Lilly wrote, *The Center of the Cyclone,* and went from there. "So I started to build one," he says. "Out of my imagination. I used to build nightclubs. I like to build things—to take shit and build it into something."

When Crash had finished the tank, he went for a float every day, about an hour at a time. "It would *beat my ass,*" he says. "I get into this thing, and it starts to *deal* with me. Like, it's showing me myself. And I'm going, *Whoa.* And that's not easy for me, because at that point in my life, I was, like, *twisted,* into a weird thing. I'd been through all this and that. Twenty-five years of drugs and, you know, *involvement.* And I got in that thing, man, and it wasn't, like, *restful* at all. It was really the strangest thing. I would do it every day. Just beat the shit out of myself for one hour."

After floating, he didn't need all the movies and music. "I would get out of that chamber and sit on the couch and I didn't have to turn nothing on," he says. "Just sit there. Like, *Whoa. So cool. I'm able to sit here, and not have to beam anything into my brain.*"

Over the course of about a year, Crash's floats stopped feeling like torture, and along the way, he says, they were a huge reason why he was able to kick narcotics. "Shored me up," he says. "Because I did have to change. I'm not the person I was. And that is why I was able to do it."

Crash felt a need to keep building these chambers and convince people to use them. He moved to Venice Beach and got a little office by the beach, and built a couple of tanks in there. He had to go through a few iterations. The first one was too small. Looked like a coffin, felt claustrophobic.

He built a big square one next, but still nobody would get in, so Crash said, "I gotta build these things *BIG!*"

What he came up with is essentially what he still uses today—about seven feet tall, eight feet long, five feet wide, with a three-by-five-foot door. It's more like a sensory deprivation closet.

Crash now has nine float tanks, two at his original spot in Venice and seven at his newer place in Westwood, where he now spends most of his time. Each tank costs him around $50,000 to build and install, and he says that's only because he has connections. The behind-the-scenes setup is stunningly elaborate, particularly his patented water disinfection filtration system, which is certified to eradicate, at minimum, 99.9 percent of contaminants—all without any chemicals. He frequently flies in an engineer from Detroit to test everything and ensure that all is working well and not going to hurt anyone.

His obsession with music feels like a lifetime ago—which, to Crash, it is. Without the chamber, maybe he and his band would've made something out of themselves, but probably not. "Best-case scenario is, we would've had some success," he says. "But then what? That would've been long gone by now. This turned out much better for me, because, you know, I'm at this age now, and I still have a future."

He says that's what he wants to give people, too—even literally. When he first opened in Venice in 2000, he charged twenty-five dollars per float, for however long people wanted to go in.

He'd let you spend the night floating. The forty dollars he charges for two hours now is unbeatable. Furthermore, Crash chafes at how most other places dilute the experience, especially those that do multiple floats without filtering the water. He rants, "Anyone who gets into one of those things is having a diminished experience. The smell is bad. They fucking stink! There were two articles in the *New York Times*, fucking both of them went into *detail* about the *smell*. Twice! You smell anything in ours? No! There is no smell. That smell is contamination. We're *clean*. It's fucking *clean*."

He points to a guy testing all the equipment. "You know how much it cost to fly him out here? Put him up in a hotel? Rent him a car?"

"Where's he from?" I ask.

"Detroit! He's here from fucking Michigan!"

"Oh, wow. I thought he was a local guy."

"No! Fuck no!"

"Nice."

"Not nice! *Re-QUIRED!*"

Talking about one particularly loathsome rival, Crash says, "The guy goes, *Ohhhh, don't like to do that, that's expensive. About every four months.* So you're thinking—so, today, you're gonna throw seven hundred dollars of your money down the drain, throw it in the toilet, right? But yesterday it was just fine to charge somebody a hundred bucks to get in there and stew around in this shit? It's criminal is what it is, and it needs to be dealt with. And that's what my job is. To make sure these fuckheads get nipped in the bud before too much longer. Even though that's not my core objective, it is indeed the result that will occur, because if not, something is going to happen to somebody in one of these things. And that's gonna fuck the whooole thing up."

Then nobody's going to trust any float tank, and Crash's great hope for humanity will be destroyed.

When you go to the Westwood location, there's a kind of entering-a-secret-world vibe.

It's a plain, nondescript glass office door tucked into the swath of stores and restaurants, beside the Corner Bakery Café. There's a small piece of laminated paper telling you how to get in: you have to press a buzzer and Crash has to unlock that door for you. Then you enter an elevator and go to the basement. A small sign in the elevator says "Float Lab," and when the door opens, another sign tells you to "enter the lounge and make yourself comfortable."

Entering said lounge feels like entering a sort of space-agey spa. Everything is black and gray and silver. A couple of black couches sprawl through the lobby, and there's Crash, sitting in a white chair behind a black-and-gray desk that holds nothing but his iPad, his MacBook Pro, lamp, and mug of coffee. Acoustic padding lines some of the walls, a throwback to Crash's studio days.

Walk into your room and you step onto a gray tile floor, a black chair and small black table to your right, a shower, open, no curtain—and the tank, which really just looks like a metallic wall with a big black door on one side. Disrobe, put the provided earplugs in, shower, then open the door and step into the darkness. The water comes up to around your shins. You lie down, and you float.

I spend the first fifteen minutes or so of my first float thinking way too much. Am I doing this right? Am I supposed to feel this? Did I ruin it by bumping into the wall? When do I start seeing things?

Avid tank users can seem downright hippie-tastic. Crash, sure. But also the guys coming through Float Lab. Earlier, in the lobby,

I got to talking with one of them who'd just finished a float. He was about Crash's age, silver beard, long gray hair, all South African accent and Zen vibes. Said he puts in about twenty-five hours a month at Float Lab, and that back in the eighties, he used another tank to do hundreds of hours a month. "It takes you all different places, man."

It's these guys who are driving floating forward. And sure, they sound silly—a few years ago, I'm embarrassed to admit, I'd probably make fun of them behind their backs—but listen to them long enough, learn enough from them, start catching glimpses of the things they call their vision, and you start to wonder if maybe we're the ones whose minds could use a little help.

And of course, we all need some help. We all have the human condition.

That said, Steph Curry is considered not only one of the best players in the NBA, but also one of the smartest. For him to buy into something like this is no small thing. The Reboot setup is different from Float Lab: individual pods, entered via a lid that can stay open if you want. The pods have lights and underwater speakers that can play music or guided meditations, and they play music to end the session. A bit more *accoutrement* than suits Crash. But Reboot tanks *are* the offspring of Crash's concept, as the man who founded Reboot, Michael Garrett, was inspired directly by Crash.

At some point during my float, I feel like I've been in there all day.

At first, I feel sort of the way Alipour and lots of other reporters seemed to feel about Float Lab—sort of arm's length, tongue-in-cheek, *Oh, this is sorta silly.*

But then everything sort of melts together. My thoughts, breathing, heartbeat. I really feel nothing. Sometimes I feel like I've fallen asleep, but I can't tell for sure.

I definitely fall out of time. A buddy of mine will later tell me his two hours felt like fifteen minutes. Fifteen minutes feels like two hours to me, and two hours feels like it could easily be half the day. I wander through my past, memories passing like full days, the way dreams feel.

I think over and over about how, during my bad times, I so often felt like I was this burden on everyone around me, and that maybe they'd all be better off if I wasn't there to burden them—if I disappeared.

I feel a kind of panic.

But then I feel euphoria.

I feel what I've heard several people say: There seems to be a specific reason why we are so acutely attuned to our feelings and our senses—we are *such* sensory creatures. I feel how fantastic it is to be a human being, to have ever gotten to play. Not just to play a sport, not just to play baseball, but just to *play*.

I understand the hippies.

I see my wife and my son dancing.

Then I see dragons. Neon indigo dragons, roaring around me. That's frustrating, at least at first, until they talk to me. Then they say something like, *Everyone has us, and we're the good dragons, here to help you fight the real monster, like in that movie you're trying to force on your son, about how to train your dragon.*

I didn't know what to make of the dragons at first, but later, given some time to process and go further down the rabbit hole that is This Stuff, I understand. First, they are not unique to me. We all have them. Sometimes, they go bad, but more often than not, the dragons in us are just neglected and misunderstood, and they behave accordingly.

Second, whatever we are, whatever our problems, however difficult life can be, whatever the goals of God or whatever it is that put us here, however crazy we become, it's still good to be here. Given the choice between being nothing versus being something, maybe we want a break to just float in nothingness, a little time *being* nothing—but it is so much better to be someone, to be something. To exist.

Lying there in the dark seeing visions and thinking about what they mean, I have another thought: when we watch our favorite athletes perform, whether it's some Herculean feat, or when we see two big football players collide, or two fighters do battle in a way that makes us writhe in our seats, or watch a man fall from space and live to tell about it, then we are bearing witness to a sort of vision . . . we are watching the payoff of someone's utmost effort to bring forth a vision of their own, a vision of utmost importance to their own heart and mind.

What I mean is, we're not *just* watching a game—or, if we are the players, we're not just playing one. People great at sport are simply people who have done what we're all trying to do: get the most out of their lives and abilities.

When athletes do great things, their feats are visions of what we as human beings are capable of, physical manifestations of battles won and lost with their own mind dragons.

We all have them—and we can all do something about them.

Now I'm not floating in space but falling through it. I see stars, and then the stars fade, and I see a giant neon-blue sphere. Earth. Or at least I think it's Earth. It's somewhere. The dragons are back and they are flying with me, toward Earth or wherever, like they have something they want me to see. These things we all want, this world we imagine, the peace we need—is it really so much more impossible for us to reach than for an Olympian to earn gold?

Then I see a spaceman, jumping from the stratos. It might

be Fearless Felix but I can't quite tell. Then there are more, and more and more and more, until there are so many of us I can't count everyone, all of us falling through space. And then I'm not so sure we're falling at all. We might be riding dragons. We might be flying.

Epilogue: The Results

"So, you getting what you needed, mate?"

I'm sitting in the middle of Red Bull North America's Santa Monica office, sipping on an espresso and exchanging jabbery rambles with Andy Walshe about all of This Stuff. The time moves toward five o'clock, and people are packing up for the day—and then there is a chorus of groans and bitter laughter, followed by a lot of people wishing each other good luck.

For the first time in weeks, it's raining in Los Angeles. Oil will make the roads slick, and traffic will be even more awful than usual. In a couple hours, a fifteen-mile drive downtown will take me an hour and a half.

For now, though, I don't care, and Walshe doesn't seem to care, either, both of us raving away about all This Stuff. Imagining the way This Stuff will move forward and reshape the world and the very meaning of what it is to be a human being feels like waking up in a lucid dream. That reshaping seems inevitable, whether in the forms I found over the past couple years, or something else entirely.

In other words, where This Stuff will take us is anybody's guess. As Mike Gervais bluntly puts it, "We're still light-years away from where this is all going."

It's not impossible that at some point in the not-too-distant future, we will be able to enter a training simulation sort of like in the movie *The Matrix*, with our brains on full display while we work, allowing us to make easy adjustments in real time. *Future Us* will likely look back on *Present Us* with pity.

And better yet, the more This Stuff shows us our brains and their errors for what they really are, the stigma surrounding mental needs will keep fading away, letting all of us breathe a little easier, and be less afraid. Last year, Brandon Marshall told the *Guardian*, "Where we're at today is where the cancer and HIV community was 20–25 years ago." In June 2016, ESPN ran a prominent feature about a young man who quit playing college football in order to treat his clinical depression, and the reporters rightly treated him like a hero—a big step in a much-needed direction. In September 2016, when Ohio State football coach Urban Meyer came forward with his story, it touched a nerve deep and raw throughout the world of sports; he received countless hundreds of e-mails and phone calls from coaches and athletes like him, saying that they were so glad to realize they were not alone.

And it seems like all of This is moving at light speed. After all, it's only been about fifteen years since Dr. Michael Merzenich showed that we could change our physical brains at all, and it took *him* more than twenty years to convince the world of that. Rewiring the global human consciousness takes an almost supernatural effort.

Plus, when it comes to This Stuff, even the smartest people in the world are feeling their way through the dark, like all of us. And we're learning new things seemingly every day. For instance, in late 2016, a team of neuroscientists discovered one hundred new regions of the brain. One *hundred*.

This is cause for excitement and concern as we hurtle toward that question mark on the wall in the Red Bull High Performance lab hall. "Everyone has an angle," Walshe says. "And you know, people build an angle for two reasons. One, it's their work and the direction life has taken them. Or two, which unfortunately is a problem with our industry, there's money to be made. If you have *theeeeeee* angle that no one else has, then you can charge a lot of money, and that's the biggest issue I see in our space. It's the snake oil. Because it's complex.

"Of course, we'd like to be able to say, *Hey, you practice this much, you train this hard, you get this psychology right, you have the right tech, you eat well, you have great doctors around you, your world off the court is as good as your world on the court, you understand all the opportunities in terms of who you are and what you're about creatively, spiritually, and humanly, and then you'll win*—but we'd be lying. I believe that all *will* help. But if you ask *anybody* in our business, at some point the reason one person stands on top of the podium, and the other's alone back in the hotel room . . . we fucking have no clue.

"I think that's the global conversation. Many people doing *deep* work in *many* areas that we're all playing in, and I think you've gotta step back, and say, *Hey, what's the contribution to the greater understanding?* And through that, you can leverage something extraordinary. But holy shit, if it's a definitive answer you're looking for, we're not gonna be able to give you that. Nobody can. We have to be very cautious of saying that *this* is the answer, versus *that*, you know? Our position is always, 'This is *a* solution that has been found effective in this particular situation.' We're always very mindful of not committing too hard. We are committed to pushing the *edge* hard, but also explaining to people that, when we are in a complex environment like the human system, in a topic that is as far out, as extraordinarily diverse and complicated as human performance is, even if we know a lot, we know one percent of what's knowable."

I laugh without meaning to, stunned and humbled by what he just said. After years of searching, after my own pathological quest for answers and my obsession with all this "next-level shit" . . . I've just been told that the smartest people in the world know *1 percent* of what's knowable. And I feel like I might know 1 percent of that 1 percent.

Walshe and I pause, taking a breather. People gather at the exit, preparing for a dicey journey home. Los Angeles needed the rain, but it's going to cause some headaches at first.

"Man," I say. "Sometimes this feels like exploring deep space."

"Right!" Walshe says, grinning big and throwing up his hands. "So, fucking jump on for the ride, everyone. Let's go!"

A few days later, I drive with my wife from San Diego to Mesa, Arizona, through red deserts and cliffs that look and feel more like Mars than Earth, and then I meet with Leslie Sherlin. After we talk for a few hours, he offers to train me the way he trains his athletes.

He hooks my brain up, and then I am using my mind to fly a spaceship.

I'm rusty. It's been a few months since Dan Chartier did my first EEG assessment, and I've spent so much time digging through all of This Stuff that I haven't gotten as much EEG training as I want. Sherlin pushes me and challenges me, reminding me of my old strength and conditioning sessions. At one point I'm struggling, and the spaceship comes to a complete stop.

Like any good coach, Sherlin nails the problem: "You're a momentum guy, right? Once you get going, you're good, but when something interrupts it, or blocks it, or hits a barrier, you're like, *Crap, I gotta start over, from the beginning.*"

By now, I have seen so much Stuff, and yet I remain amazed at how well it works, and how good people like Sherlin are at using it.

"Make it a little easier on yourself," he says. "When you feel it get harder, what I want you to do is try to just roll with it. The reason it's getting hard is because you're making really good progress, right? Reframe. Reset."

We do a few more sessions. I have some bumpy moments, and I feel that old familiar tension rise; the mind dragons stir. But then I ride them. I breathe like Pierre Beauchamp taught me. I remember to have fun with it. And then I slip into the greatest headspace, feeling zoned in, and relaxed, and at peace. I feel . . . clear.

"Outstanding," Sherlin says. "Remember that feeling."

And then Sherlin says something I wasn't sure I'd ever hear. He said, "Your brain looks good."

Wherever This Stuff is taking us, it's really the same place we've always wanted to be.

In the deserts of ancient North Africa, tribes gathered at night for sacred moonlight dances. These often lasted for hours, until dawn. This was their way of expressing themselves, together.

But sometimes one of the dancers would start moving and singing in a way that transcended the rest. The tribesmen would gather around, drawn by them, and begin to chant. *All-ah, All-ah, All-ah.*

God. God. God.

Over the course of history and as a result of many migrations, the chant made its way into Europe. You would recognize it today as *Ole! Ole-Ole-Ole!!! Ole! Ole!!!*

Ancient humans believed sports to be a gift from the gods, given to us for some divine purpose. The ancient Greeks used athletic competition as a means to test the respectability and capability and strength of their leaders. They also treated athletic contests as offerings to the gods, a way to channel some of their aggression and passion into entertainment, into something of value and worth: a display of what human beings are capable of. They saw participation in sports, whether as athlete or witness, as something that educated, enriched, and even freed the soul.

Hit Earth with an asteroid tomorrow, and we will play in the wreckage.

Our genes must hold some ancient, unconscious knowledge of how good sports are for us. Remember: we have not only one brain, but several, all competing with each other all the time, and it's a fight totally different and so much harder than anything we'll face on the outside. To compete in sport is, after all, also to compete against yourself. Beyond sports, so much that leaves us defeated comes from within.

Something in us craves those transcendent moments, and not only as performers, but as witnesses. Simply put, feeling *awe* like that makes us better, and not just in an abstract sense: when we experience awe—defined as "that sense of wonder we feel in the presence of something so vast it transcends our understanding of the world"—whether in religion, art, music, or something else, it unleashes a cascade of neurochemical reactions that transform us. Awe makes us want to bond more closely with those around us, reduces inflammation, lifts us out of bad moods, and makes us more empathetic, trusting, and kind.

Some say that awe lies at the heart of all religions, and sport is easily one of the world's favorite religious practices. Whether watching or playing, we are all in search of that great *Ole!*

Those moments of awe in sports are maybe the best, purest moments human beings experience. Great movies and music can feel as good as the best drugs, but they also have writers who pore over every word, and small armies of people engineering the heck out of them. But in sports, there's no director yelling cut, no record producer tweaking the sound levels, no photographer's assistant getting the lighting just so. In sports, there are no second takes.

There is only the moment, and then it is gone.

The only other place like it is life itself.

And I think those perfect moments feel sent by God because maybe something in us knows that at any given moment, our brains will sabotage us. Perfection is scientifically impossible. Imperfection is like a permanent glitch in our system that cannot be repaired, or predicted, or prevented. No matter how masterful we become at a given task, no matter how mentally strong we become, sometimes, for absolutely no known reason whatsoever, the neurons in our brain will simply misfire.

That's why Steph Curry can be the greatest shooter in the history of basketball and still brick a wide-open jumper.

That's why no matter what I tried, I couldn't throw the ball back to the pitcher.

That's why no matter how enlightened we become, no matter how much we learn to engineer our minds, we will still screw up. We are all destined for imperfection. We are all fated to be victims of the human condition.

There's this park around the corner from my house that my son, Jonah, loves. He runs around, we kick soccer balls, he throws baseballs, he climbs ladders and dives down slides. Sometimes I forget he's only two years old.

The park has a little baseball field, too, and one day Katie and I and our son were playing baseball with this fat orange bat and little purple plastic baseball. At first he was hitting the ball but then he wanted to run the bases, which really meant just run all over the place, as toddlers do. And then he wanted to chase balls that *we* hit.

So often I forget to just enjoy these moments. As good as my brain might look now, I can still be a self-absorbed jerk, and get too focused on my own work instead of my time with my family. But sometimes, I am also way better than I ever thought I could be. More often every passing month, I feel like myself again.

Katie and I took turns tossing the ball to each other, hitting soft liners out into the grass, and our son chased them down.

He's growing up so fast. Soon he'll be asking for advice, and one day he might even want to go pro in some sport himself. But now I know what I'll tell him. I'll tell him that wanting to go pro is great, so go for it, and working hard is great, so work hard, and wanting to be perfect is great, so try to be perfect. I'll tell him about This Stuff, and we will learn more about it all, together, as it evolves. But I'll also tell him that for all of this futuristic technology, for all of this deep science, for all of this awesome Stuff, there is one overlooked secret greater than the rest. I'll tell him, *Whatever you do, remember what I forgot. Remember to have fun.*

Whether playing sports, or watching them, or just going through life, when we chase perfect moments, when we try to experience something beyond the world as we know it, we'll never quite get there if we're not having fun. In the complex production that is our brain and that is this life, fun is the oil in the engine.

Katie and I kept taking turns hitting because our son just wanted to chase the ball. And, as tends to occur with us, things turned competitive; we started trying to strike each other out.

Inevitably, my last turn hitting, Katie wound up and blazed one in there—and I actually swung and missed.

In the past that would have stressed me out. Yes, even though we were playing *Wiffle ball* with an *orange plastic bat* and *purple plastic ball* with our two-year-old son, I still would have had this irrational need to not look like I sucked, *to prove myself.*

I know. It's ridiculous.

But today was different.

Because today, I just laughed.

And I swear, I could feel the air change around us, becoming lighter and clearer, and within it we all felt more free.

"Hit ball, Daddy!" Jonah said.

I picked up the ball and threw it back to Katie and said, "Try that again."

She grinned back, then wound up, and I geared up to swing, to really show her who's boss, and—she lobbed one in there, and I was laughing so hard I swung way too soon and barely tipped the ball with the end of the bat.

"Strike two," she said.

"Pressure, pressure," I said, picking up the ball and tossing it back to her.

"Daddy, hit *ball*!"

One more windup, and then Katie threw the ball as hard as she could, and I took my last swing of the day. And then what happened next had us all laughing even harder, for all kinds of reasons.

I hit it on the barrel. Jonah started to chase the ball, but then threw up his hands and said, "Oh?!" He didn't know where the ball had gone.

The ball had gone everywhere. The ball was not a ball anymore. It was scattered around the field, shattered into a dozen pieces.

Acknowledgments

Without you, Katie, there would be no book. There would be no me. Thank you, thank you, thank you, for putting up with me all these years and riding out my waves of crazy with me. I still believe in God because of you, and how you showed me what love is.

Albert and Susie, thank you for being amazing parents to Katie, and in-laws to me, and Papa and Gigi to the kid, and especially for helping Katie and the kid so much when I have to leave town for work on these crazy quests for answers. Couldn't do it without you. I hope you know how much I appreciate you.

My agent, Eric Lupfer at WME, thank you for taking me on as a client, and for your genius insight that sold this book in the first place. I was like, *How about a book about fear and sports?* and you were all like, *Well fear's kind of a bummer but maybe someone is studying the minds of athletes and that could be interesting?* and well, now here we are.

My first editor at Dey Street, Denise Oswald, thank you for wanting this book. I'm sorry you didn't get to see it through, but I'm happy you got promoted and I know you're kicking butt on other rad books.

My new editor at Dey Street, Matthew Daddona, thank you for believing in this as much as Denise did, and for all of your hard work and good talks along the way.

My friend and consultant, Glenn, thank you for showing me where I kept letting Migsby get in my way. "Be simple. Be clear." And "Good is better than perfect, especially since perfect is impossible." I think someone else said that second one but thanks for pointing it out. Oh, and for letting me crash at your place and for sharing your chili and whiskey.

Jack Cassidy, thank you for your fantastic fact-checking.

And other thank-yous to . . .

Mom and Dad, for everything you have given me.

My brothers and sisters—all four of you, Kramer, Kara, Logan, Heidi—for being great aunts and uncles and for just being you, in all your unique ways. Even if it's not always obvious, when I write, I'm always thinking of all of you.

My good friend Brandon Hassell, for showing me what it means to simply be a good man. You're gonna be such a good dad.

My college journalism adviser, Rick Stewart, for—among many, many other things—first showing me that this is something I could actually do. I'm still not sure you know how much you helped me in college, during what was a very volatile time in my life.

My many other good friends, too. You know who you are.

Those of you who also read the book and provided those unbelievably kind early reviews—Lars Anderson, Brin-Jonathan Butler, Kate Fagan, Will Leitch, Don Van Natta, Jeff Pearlman, Peter Richmond. Our conversations about the book, however in-depth or brief, helped me more than you'll know, even if only to provide some peace that I didn't totally waste my time on this crazy quest the last few years.

Team Omega/Halfway House/Edwards, because sometimes it

feels good to just go play a dumb, fun game like softball with a great bunch of guys. The winning doesn't hurt.

Starbucks, for producing the countless gallons of coffee, tea, and doughnuts I consumed over the past few years.

Everyone who actually did talk to me for this book, particularly Dan Chartier, Mike Gervais, and Leslie Sherlin, for all of our conversations beyond the scope of this book, and for showing me how my brain can actually look good.

There are way too many more people I probably should thank here. I hope you all know who you are. If you're not listed here, I owe you a drink.

Finally, everyone who is doing good, deep work in this space of figuring out the brain and putting that knowledge out into the world for the rest of us. I admire the heck out of you, and owe you my life. I hope I didn't desecrate your beautiful work in trying to write about it using my meager brain. Please let me know if I messed something up, and I'll do my best to correct the error. At the very least, though, I hope you enjoyed the read. I hope I've done some small part in helping the world by sharing your work, and I can't wait to see what you will show us next.

Notes and Sources

I'm not going to name most of the obvious sports sources because this list is already too long, and most are referenced directly in the text.

These lists will make up about half of my sources, give or take—for every interview or article listed here I had at least a few more—but I think this will give you enough to know where the stuff in the book comes from, and where to start looking if you want to explore some more.

(In the case of online references, all dates provided below are the dates the web page was last updated as of this writing.)

General Selected Bibliography

Here are some select articles and books that provided a solid foundation for writing about all of This Stuff:

Amthor, Frank. *Neuroscience for Dummies.* Mississauga, Ontario, Canada: John Wiley & Sons Canada.

Babiloni, Claudio, et al. "Neural efficiency of experts' brain during judgment of actions: A high-resolution EEG study in elite and amateur karate athletes." *Behavioural Brain Research.* November 3, 2009.

Baumeister, Jochen. "Cortical activity of skilled performance in a complex sports-related motor task." *Journal of Applied Physiology.* July 8, 2008.

Baumeister, Jochen, et al. "Brain activity in goal-directed movements in a real compared to a virtual environment using the Nintendo Wii." *Neuroscience Letters.* June 18, 2010.

Boecker, H. "A role of the basal ganglia and midbrain nuclei for initiation of motor sequences." *NeuroImage*. October 16, 2007.

Bronson, Po, and Ashley Merryman. *Top Dog*. New York: Hachette, 2013.

Carter, Rita. *Mapping the Mind*. Los Angeles: University of California Press, 2010.

Cortright, Brant. *The Neurogenesis Diet & Lifestyle*. Mill Valley, CA: Psyche Media, 2015.

Coyle, Daniel. *The Talent Code*. New York: Random House, 2010.

Csikszentmihalyi, Mihaly. *Flow*. New York: Harper Perennial, 2008.

Doidge, Norman. *The Brain That Changes Itself*. New York: Penguin, 2007.

Eagleman, David. *The Brain*. New York: Pantheon Books, 2015.

Epstein, David. *The Sports Gene*. New York: Penguin, 2014.

Faubert, Jocelyn. "Professional athletes have extraordinary skills for rapidly learning complex and neutral dynamic visual scenes." *Scientific Reports*. January 31, 2013.

Fichetti, Mark. "Computers versus Brains." *Scientific American*. October 12, 2011.

Fitzgerald, Matt. *How Bad Do You Want It?* Boulder, CO: Velo Press, 2015.

Gaoxia Wei, and Jeng Luo. "Sports expert's motor imagery: Functional imaging of professional motor skills and simple motor skills." *Brain Research*. August 15, 2009.

Gibb, Barry J. *The Rough Guide to the Brain*. London, England: Rough Guides Ltd., 2012.

Gordon, Dan. *Your Brain on Cubs*. New York: Dana Press, 2008.

Jackson, Susan A., and Mihaly Csikszentmihalyi. *Flow in Sports*. Champaign, IL: Human Kinetics, 1999.

Kahneman, Daniel. *Thinking, Fast and Slow*. New York: Farrar, Straus and Giroux, 2013.

Kaku, Michio. *Future of the Mind*. New York: Anchor Books, 2014.

Kim, Jingu. "Athletes in a Slump: Neurophysiological Evidence from Frontal Theta Activity." Maryland Institute of Research (MIR). January 2014.

Koppel, Barbara S. "The Neuroscience Behind Sports." *Neurology Today.* September 4, 2008.

Kotler, Steven. *The Rise of Superman.* New York: New Harvest, 2014.

Marchant, Jo. *Cure.* New York: Crown Publishers, 2016.

Matta, Eduardo, et al. "Neuroscience of Exercise: From Neurobiology Mechanisms to Mental Health." *Neuropsychobiology.* September 28, 2012.

Medina, John. *Brain Rules.* Seattle, WA: Pear Press, 2008.

Milton, John. "The brain and brawn of athletic performance." http://faculty.jsd.claremont.edu/jmilton/reprints/chicago_05.pdf. January 12, 2005.

Milton, John, et al. "The mind of expert motor performance is cool and focused." *Neuroimage.* April 1, 2007.

Mumford, George. *The Mindful Athlete.* Berkeley, CA: Parallax Press, 2015.

Nakata, Hiroki, et al. "Characteristics of the athletes' brain: Evidence from neurophysiology and neuroimaging." *Brain Research Reviews.* November 26, 2009.

Newberg, Andrew, and Mark Robert Waldman. *How God Changes Your Brain.* New York: Ballantine Books, 2010.

Oishi, Kazuo, and Takashi Maeshima. "Autonomic Nervous System Activities During Motor Imagery in Elite Athletes." *Journal of Clinical Neurophysiology.* June 2004.

Ramachandran, V.S. *The Tell-Tale Brain.* New York: W. W. Norton & Company, 2011.

Robbins, Jim. *A Symphony in the Brain.* New York: Grove Press, 2008.

Schwartz, Jeffrey M., and Sharon Begley. *The Mind and the Brain.* New York: HarperCollins, 2002.

Snow, Shane. *Smartcuts.* New York: Harper Business, 2014.

Vorhauser-Smith, Sylvia. "The Neuroscience of Performance: PageUp People White Paper." PageUpPeople.com. June 2012.

Wolf, Sebastian, et al. "Motor skill failure or flow-experience? Functional brain asymmetry and brain connectivity in elite and amateur table tennis players." *Biological Psychology.* September 23, 2014.

Notes and Select Sources by Chapter

PROLOGUE

I'm very grateful to Andy Walsh at Red Bull, who was one of the chief people in sports who helped me feel like this was a topic and book worth pursuing. I was so glad when he actually showed up in that lobby that day. I'd spoken with him on the phone a few times before, e-mailed a bit, and then he was so gracious he spent a whole day with me talking about This Stuff—stepping away for a meeting here and there—in the middle of a time that was busy as "all bloody hell."

Michael Gervais spent hours upon hours on the phone with me, usually with one or both of us in an airport across the country from each other, and one time while I was driving through a blizzard.

Herb Yoo, formerly of Nike before founding Senaptec with Joe Bingold, also spent hours on the phone with me and was one of the very first people I spoke to about any of This Stuff.

CHAPTER 1

"Lotus Pose on Two," the Seattle Seahawks profile in the August 13, 2013 *ESPN The Magazine* mentioned in this chapter, was one of the first of many articles to show me just how athletes could be using This Stuff.

Leslie Sherlin spent hours on the phone with me, too, and invited me out to his office in Phoenix. I learned a lot from him.

Some of the books I read that provided an invaluable springboard for studying This Stuff were *The Brain That Changes Itself* by Norman Doidge, *Flow* by Mihaly Csikszentmihalyi, and *The Rise of Superman* by Steven Kotler.

CHAPTER 2

There's no way for me to adequately thank Dan Chartier for the many, many hours he spent talking with me, hooking my brain up, and then helping me figure it out. If you're curious about EEG training, or simply want a good man to talk to about your psychological needs, visit Life Quality Resources in Raleigh, N.C. Their website is lifequalityresources.org.

Leslie Sherlin was also an invaluable resource for this chapter.

Also invaluable was the book *A Symphony in the Brain* by Jim Robbins, who was also so kind as to spend some time talking with me on the phone.

CHAPTER 3

Once again, Sherlin came up big for me for this chapter, as did Andy Walshe and Michael Gervais. Sherlin's company, SenseLabs, also provided me with several videos, papers, and other documents, by e-mail and via their website, that were very useful.

Dan Chartier was also a critical resource for this chapter.

CHAPTER 4

Gervais was big for this chapter, as well as the following select sources:

Amroth, Frank. *Neuroscience for Dummies.*
Carter, Rita. *Mapping the Mind.*
Eagleman, David. *The Brain.*
Eliasmith, Chris, et al. "A Large-Scale Model of a Functioning Brain." *Science.* November 2012.
Fichetti, Mark. "Computers versus Brains." *Scientific American.* October 12, 2011.
Gibb, Barry J. *A Rough Guide to the Brain.*
Muller, Daphne. "Your Brain Isn't a Computer—It's a Quantum Field." BigThink.com. September 21, 2015.
Roenigk, Alyssa. "Lotus Pose on Two." *ESPN The Magazine.* August 21, 2013.

CHAPTER 5

This chapter benefited from interviews with Andy Walsh and Michael Gervais, not to mention Dan Chao, the founder of Halo Sport, and Wes Clapp and Brian Miller, founders of NeuroScouting, all of whom are so smart and who were so fun to talk with about This Stuff.

And I can't forget Oliver Marmol, the former pro ballplayer turned coach and "neuro" geek like me. He was brave to share his story so openly with me. I greatly appreciate it, and I'm sure many others will, too.

Also, I am hugely grateful to the hard work of many who came before me, as I built this chapter in large part from a cornucopia of sources. Among them:

Archer, Dale. "How ADHD Puts Athletes in the Zone." *Forbes*. July 16, 2014.

Bieler, Des. "Simone Biles not 'ashamed' to say she has ADHD after anti-doping database hack." *Washington Post*. September 13, 2016.

Breslow, Jason M. "76 of 79 Deceased NFL Players Found to Have Brain Disease." PBS.org. September 30, 2014.

Ching, Justin. "Mental health issues a huge challenge for NCAA in regard to student-athletes." FoxSports.com. March 25, 2015.

Daugherty, Paul. "Reds' Votto finds strength to battle mental health stigma in locker room." *Cincinnati Enquirer*. June 23, 2009.

Delsohn, Steve. "OTL: Belcher's brain had CTE signs." ESPN.com. September 30, 2014.

GoPro. "GoPro: Red Bull Stratos—The Full Story." YouTube. January 31, 2014.

Harrell, Illya. "Joey Votto Makes His Personal Demons Public." Bleacher Report. June 24, 2009.

Hughes, Lynette, and Gerard Leavey. "Setting the bar: athletes and vulnerability to mental illness." *British Journal of Psychiatry*. February 2012.

Keown, Tim. "Discussing mental illness." ESPN.com. May 16, 2013.

McRae, Donald. "Felix Baumgartner: 'I hope I can make fear cool.'" *Guardian*. November 2, 2012.

New, Jake. "Study: 1 in 4 College Athletes Show Signs of Depression." *Inside Higher Ed*. January 28, 2016.

Red Bull. "Red Bull Stratos—World Record Freefall." YouTube. October 15, 2012.

RedBullStratos.com.

Rhoden, William C. "With No One Looking, a Hurt Stays Hidden." *New York Times*. October 29, 2012.

Roenigk, Alyssa. "Doctors say late BMX legend Dave Mirra had CTE." ESPN.com. May 24, 2016.

Shergold, Adam. "Supersonic skydiver Felix Baumgartner found guilty of punching Greek lorry driver in road rage incident." *Daily Mail*. November 6, 2012.

Smith, Marty. "How do you cope when it's over?" ESPN.com. May 11, 2012.

Sneed, Brandon. "I'm Not the Lone Wolf." *B/R Mag* at Bleacher Report. September 13, 2016.

Streep, Peg. "The Communal Narcissist: Another Wolf Wearing a Sheep Outfit." *Psychology Today.* May 24, 2016.

Tarkan, Laurie. "Athletes' Injuries Go Beyond the Physical." *New York Times.* September 26, 2000.

Troncale, Joseph. "Your Lizard Brain: The Limbic System and Brain Functioning." *Psychology Today.* April 22, 2014.

Wiese-Bjornstal, Diane M., et al. "An integrated model of response to sport injury: Psychological and sociological dynamics." *Applied Sport Psychology.* January 14, 2008.

Wolanin, et al. "Prevalence of clinically elevated depressive symptoms in college athletes and differences by gender and sport." *British Journal of Sports Medicine.* December 7, 2015.

CHAPTER 6

Once again, I owe a debt of gratitude to Andy Walshe, Michael Gervais, Oliver Marmol, Dan Chartier, and Leslie Sherlin for their input on the matters in this chapter.

In addition, some select sources produced by brilliant, hardworking, bold people:

Acharya, Sourya, and Samarth Shukla. "Mirror neurons: Enigma of the metaphysical modular brain." *Journal of Natural Science, Biology, and Medicine.* July 2012.

Bergland, Christopher. "5 Neuroscience Based Ways to Clear Your Mind." *Psychology Today.* April 15, 2015.

———. "Why Does Overthinking Cause Athletes to Choke?" *Psychology Today.* August 8, 2013.

Bieler, Des. "Simone Biles not 'ashamed' to say she has ADHD after anti-doping database hack." *Washington Post.* September 13, 2016.

Broadway, Bill. "Is the Capacity for Spirituality Determined by Our Brain Chemistry?" *Washington Post.* November 13, 2004.

Carey, Benedict. "Do You Believe in Magic?" *New York Times.* January 23, 2007.

———. "Long-Awaited Medical Study Questions the Power of Prayer." *New York Times.* March 31, 2006.

Cohen, Julie. "Overthinking Can Be Detrimental to Athletic Performance." *Journal of Neuroscience.* August 7, 2013.

Curtis, Ramsden. *Emergency and Trauma Nursing.* Sydney, Australia: Elsevier, 2007.

Davidson, Richard. "Buddha's Brain: Neuroplasticity and Meditation." *IEEE Signal Process Magazine.* September 2008.

Effron, Lauren. "Michael Jordan, Kobe Bryant's Meditation Coach on How to Be 'Flow Ready' and Get in the Zone." ABCNews.com. April 6, 2016.

FocusBand.com.

Gallahan, William, et al. "An analysis of the placebo effect in Crohn's disease over time." *Ailment Pharmacological Therapy.* January 2010.

Geirland, John. "Buddha on the Brain." *Wired.* February 1, 2016.

Gilsinan, Kathy. "The Brains of the Buddhists." *Atlantic.* July 4, 2015.

Gladding, Rebecca. "This Is Your Brain on Meditation." *Psychology Today.* May 22, 2013.

Goodwin, John. *Unsolved: The World of the Unknown.* New York: Doubleday, 1976.

Goudreau, Jenna. "Superstitions and Magical Thinking." *Forbes.* April 13, 2012.

Hagerty, Barbara Bradley. "Prayer May Reshape Your Brain . . . And Your Reality." NPR.com. May 20, 2009.

Hamer, Dean. *The God Gene.* New York: Anchor Books, 2005.

Harvard University. "Prayers Don't Help Heart Surgery Patients; Some Fare Worse When Prayed For." *Science Daily.* April 3, 2006.

Holzel, Britta K., et al. "How Does Mindfulness Meditation Work? Proposing Mechanisms of Action from a Conceptual and Neural Perspective." *Perspectives on Psychological Science.* November 2011.

Hutson, Matthew. "The Science of Superstition." *Atlantic.* March 2015.

Hyman, Ira. "Superstitions and the Super Bowl." *Psychology Today.* January 28, 2015.

Iacoboni, Marco. *Mirroring People: The New Science of How We Connect with Others.* New York: Farrar, Straus and Giroux, 2008.

Johnson, Amy. "How Understanding Neuroscience Helps Me Get Unstuck." *Schizophrenia Bulletin.* May 2015.

Kilner, J. M., and R. N. Lemon. "What We Currently Know About Mirror Neurons." *Current Biology.* December 2, 2013.

Kotler, Steven. "The Neurochemistry of Superstition." *Psychology Today.* July 26, 2008.

———. *The Rise of Superman.*

Lachmann, Suzanna. "After a One-Night Stand What Comes Next?" *Psychology Today.* April 28, 2014.

Langer, Ellen. "Mind-Set Matters: Exercise and the Placebo Effect." *Psychological Science.* February 2007.

Langone, John. "In Search of the 'God Gene.'" *New York Times.* November 2, 2004.

Lehrer, Jonah. "The Mirror Neuron Revolution: Explaining What Makes Humans Social" (interview with Marco Iacoboni). *Scientific American.*

McGreevey, Sue. "Eight weeks to a better brain." *Harvard Gazette.* January 21, 2011.

Mumford, George. *The Mindful Athlete.*

Newberg, Andrew. *How God Changes Your Brain.*

———. *Principles of Neurotheology.* Burlington, VT: Ashgate Publishing, 2010.

Nike Soccer. "Nike Soccer Presents: Pro Genius Self-Talk ft. Joe Hart." YouTube. July 5, 2016.

No author given. "Meditation improves the immune system, research shows." *Telegraph.* November 1, 2011.

OSVEA TV. "J Day routine." YouTube. March 20, 2016.

Rankin, Lissa. *Mind Over Medicine.* Carlsbad, CA: Hay House, Inc., 2014.

Reiner, Peter B. "Meditation on demand: New research reveals how meditation changes the brain." *Scientific American.* May 26, 2009.

Ricard, Matthieu, et al. "Neuroscience Reveals the Secrets of Meditation's Benefits." *Scientific American.* November 1, 2014.

Rose, Ronald. *Living Magic.* Whitefish, MT: Kessinger Publishing, 2010.

Ryan, Shane. "The Masters Retro Diary." *Grantland.* April 15, 2013.

Schafer, Scott, et al. "Conditioned placebo analgesia persists when subjects know they are receiving a placebo." *Journal of Pain.* July 2015.

Schmidt, Stefan, and Harald Walach. *Meditation—Neuroscientific Approaches and Philosophical Implications.* New York: Springer, 2014.

Shea, Christopher. "Mindful Exercise." *New York Times.* December 9, 2007.

Shipnuck, Alan. "Masters 2014: Jason Day on verge of a major breakthrough." Golf.com. April 6, 2014.

Spiegel, Alex. "Hotel Maids Challenge the Placebo Effect." NPR.com. January 3, 2008.

Staik, Athena. "Four Steps to Rewire Your Brain with Conscious-Mind Action." Psychcentral.com. January 14, 2013.

Talk of the Nation. "Neurotheology: This Is Your Brain on Religion." NPR.com. December 15, 2010.

Tracey, Irene, et al. "The Effect of Treatment Expectation on Drug Efficacy: Imaging the Analgesic Benefit of the Opioid Remifentanil." *Science Translational Medicine.* February 2011.

University of Colorado–Boulder. "Know it's a placebo? The 'medicine' could still work." Colorado.edu. July 21, 2015.

Webb, Nadia. "The Neurobiology of Bliss—Sacred and Profane." *Scientific American.* July 12, 2011.

Wilson, Russell. "One Mission." *Player's Tribune.* January 27, 2015.

Winell, Marlene. *Leaving the Fold.* Oakland, CA: New Harbinger Publications, Inc., 1994.

——. "Understanding Religious Trauma Syndrome: It's Time to Recognize It." Babcp.com (British Association for Behavioural and Cognitive Psychotherapies).

——. "Understanding Religious Trauma Syndrome: Trauma from Religion." Babcp.com.

——. "Understanding Religious Trauma Syndrome: Trauma from Leaving Religion." Babcp.com.

Winerman, Lea. "The Mind's Mirror." apa.org (American Psychological Association). October 2005.

CHAPTER 7

This chapter was built from two days spent with the far too generous, kind—and most of all, patient—Pierre Beauchamp. He also sent me home with many documents and files to read for homework.

Other select sources:

Bains, Jaideep S., et al. "Stress-related synaptic plasticity in the hypothalamus." *Nature.* June 19, 2015.

Columbia University. "History of Neuroscience." Columbia.edu. No date given.

Daemen, M.J.A.P. "The heart and the brain: an intimate and underestimated relation." *Netherlands Heart Journal.* January 3, 2013.

Harvard University. "Understanding the Stress Response." Health.harvard.edu. March 18, 2016.

Rodolfo, Kelvin. "What Is Homeostasis?" *Scientific American.* No date given.

Stanford University. "A History of the Brain." Stanford.edu. No date given.

The Editors of Encyclopaedia Britannica. "Homeostasis." Britannica.com. August 26, 2015.

The Heart Math Institute. "The Heart-Brain Connection." HeartMath.org. No date given.

CHAPTER 8

This chapter was also built from my time with Beauchamp, not to mention a day spent at the Thought Technology offices in Montreal with his cohorts Marc Saab, Larry Klein, and Hal Myers.

Also, thank you to Brendan Parsons at Neurodezign for his insight.

CHAPTER 9

Gratitude to Michael Gervais and Aubrey Marcus for their insight, and a separate, even bigger thank-you to Urban Meyer for his insight.

Other select sources:

Archer, Todd. "Jerry Jones: Ezekiel Elliott's pot dispensary visit 'just not good.'" ESPN.com. August 26, 2016.

Belin, David, Barry Everitt, et al. "Basolateral and central amygdala differentially recruit and maintain dorsolateral striatum-dependent cocaine-seeking habits." *Nature Communications.* August 10, 2015.

———. "Neural mechanisms underlying the vulnerability to develop compulsive drug-seeking habits and addiction." *Philosophical Transactions of the Royal Society B.* October 12, 2008.

Belin, David, et al. "High impulsivity predicts the switch to compulsive cocaine-taking." *Science.* June 6, 2008.

Berrendero, Fernando, et al. "Neurobiological mechanisms involved in nicotine dependence and reward: participation of the endogenous opioid system." *Neuroscience Biobehavior Review.* November 2010.

Centers for Disease Control and Prevention. "Prescription Opioid Overdose Data." CDC.gov. June 21, 2016.

Chawla, Jasvinder. "Neurological Effects of Caffeine." *Medscape.* November 11, 2015.

Drugs.com. "Oxycodone." May 20, 2016.

Freeman, Mike. "Banned but Bountiful: Marijuana Coveted by NFL Players as Invaluable Painkiller." Bleacher Report. June 30, 2015.

Gilpin, Nicholas W., and George F. Koob. "Neurobiology of Alcohol Dependence." Niaaa.nih.gov. No date given.

Gowin, Joshua. "Your Brain on Alcohol." *Psychology Today.* June 18, 2010.

Gupta, Sanjay. "Medical marijuana and the 'entourage effect.'" CNN .com. March 11, 2014.

Hampson, Aidan J., Julius Axelrod, and Maurizio Grimaldi. "Cannabinoids as Antioxidants and Neuroprotectants." Original Assignee: The United States of America as Represented by the Department of Health and Human Services. Patent US6630507 B1. October 7, 2003.

Hruby, Patrick. "American caffeine addiction races full speed ahead." *Washington Times.* January 17, 2012.

———. "The NFL's Hazy Logic on Marijuana." *Atlantic.* September 17, 2014.

Jaffe, Adi. "Alcohol, Benzos, and Opiates—Withdrawal That Might Kill You." *Psychology Today.* January 13, 2010.

Kinkhabwala, Aditi. "There's Grass on the Football Field." *Wall Street Journal.* April 23, 2010.

Lafuente, H., et al. "Cannabidoil reduces brain damage and improves functional recovery after acute hypoxia-ischemia in newborn pigs." *Pediatric Research.* September 2011.

Masters, Sam. "Cannabis 'no worse than junk food' says report." *Independent.* October 14, 2012.

McCoppin, Robert. "Ex-Bear Jim McMahon: Medical marijuana got me off narcotic pain pills." *Chicago Tribune.* January 29, 2016.

Morris News Service. "Chipper goes cold turkey." *Augusta Chronicle.* May 25, 2001.

National Institute on Drug Abuse. "DrugFacts: Heroin." Drugabuse .gov. October 2014.

Onnit.com.

Persad, Leanna. "Energy Drinks and the Neurophysiological Impact of Caffeine." *Frontiers in Neuroscience.* October 21, 2011.

Psychology Today. "Nicotine." No date given.

Sneed, Brandon. "I'm Not the Lone Wolf." *B/R Mag* at Bleacher Report. September 13, 2016.

Snyder, Deron, and Bill Koenig. "Baseball's tobacco war." *USA Today.* April 8, 1998.

Szalavitz, Maia. "Can You Get Over an Addiction?" *New York Times.* June 25, 2016.

Tobacco-Related Disease Research Program. "Neuroscience of Nicotine Addiction and Treatment." TRDRP.org. No date given.

University of Cambridge. "Cocaine addiction: Scientists discover 'back door' into the brain." ScienceDaily. January 12, 2016.

Wagner, James. "With grinding schedule, more and more major leaguers are consuming energy drinks to help." *Washington Post.* July 8, 2013.

CHAPTER 10

Daniel Chao, Andy Walshe, and Greg Appelbaum provided valuable insight for this chapter, as did Thync CEO Jamie Tyler.

Other select sources:

Archer, Todd. "Jerry Jones: Ezekiel Elliott's pot dispensary visit 'just not good.'" ESPN.com. August 26, 2016.

Cogiamanian, Filippo, et al. "Improved isometric force endurance after transcranial direct current stimulation over the human motor cortical areas." *European Journal of Neuroscience.* July 2007.

Cox, David. "Dean Karnazes: the man who can run for ever." *Guardian.* August 30, 2013.

Facebook.com/JoshNorman24.

Facebook.com/Thync.

Haloneuro.com.

Hutchinson, Alex. "For the Golden State Warriors, Brain Zapping Could Provide an Edge." *New Yorker.* June 15, 2016.

———. "Your Body on Brain Doping." *Outside.* August 2, 2014.

Hoppes, Nate. "How Does the Brain of an Elite Athlete Work?" RedBull.com. June 12, 2014.

NeuroPace.com.

Okano, Alexandre, et al. "Brain stimulation modulates the autonomic nervous system, rating of perceived exertion and performance during maximal exercise." *British Journal of Sports Medicine.* September 2015.

Ranville, Anthony. "Thync—Josh Norman with Business Insider—Social Video." Vimeo. August 2016.

Red Bull. "Endurance: Exploring the Limits and Potential." RedBull.com. July 2014.

Rose, Brent. "Can This New Gadget Give You Mental Superpowers?" GQ.com. September 23, 2015.

Stokel-Walker, Chris. "5 Bizarre and Scary Historical Headache Cures." Mental Floss. September 13, 2013.

Taylor, Tom. "Mind over matter: Ultrarunner Dean Karnazes's brain-training device." *Sports Illustrated.* September 29, 2015.

Thync.com

Underwood, Emily. "Cadaver study casts doubts on how zapping brain may boost mood, relieve pain." *Science.* April 20, 2016.

CHAPTER 11

David Poole spent hours on the phone with me for this chapter, and I am grateful.

Other select sources:

Colzato, Lorenza S., et al. "More attentional focusing through binaural beats: evidence from the global-local task." *Psychological Research.* November 26, 2015.

McGill University. "Anxiety neurotransmitters." thebrain.mcgill.ca. No date given.

NuCalm.com.

Ross, Bernhard. "Binaural Beats, Brain Rhythms, and Binaural Hearing." Neuroscience.stanford.edu. October 10, 2014.

Royal Netherlands Academy of Arts and Sciences. "H. W. Dove (1803–1879)."

Watanabe, Masahito, et al. "GABA and GABA Receptors in the Central Nervous System and Other Organs." *International Review of Cytology*. Amsterdam, Netherlands: Academic Press, 2002.

PART THREE INTRODUCTION

I learned a great deal from conversations with Jason Sada and Brandon Payne.

Additional select sources:

Amos, Jonathan. "Why top sports stars might have 'more time' on the ball." BBC.com. September 5, 2012.

Dutton, Kevin. "Do You Have to Be a Psychopath to Be a Great Athlete?" BigThink.com. August 13, 2016.

Gladwell, Malcolm. *Outliers*. New York: Little, Brown and Company, 2008.

Hagura, Nobuhiro, et al. "Ready steady slow: action preparation slows the subject's passage of time." *Proceedings of the Royal Society B*. September 5, 2012.

MacLaughlin, Dan. TheDanPlan.com.

O'Hanlon, Ryan. "Time May Slow Down for Elite Athletes." *Outside*. September 6, 2012.

CHAPTER 12

Once again, Brandon Payne was huge for me this chapter. Loved thinking out loud with him about all of This Stuff, particularly his work with Steph Curry. Smart guy, fun to talk with.

Mark Hallis at FITLIGHT was also great fun to talk with and learn from.

Other select sources:

FITLIGHTTraining.com.

George, Thomas. "PRO Football: Strength and Conditioning Coaches: The Force Is with Them." *New York Times*. June 27, 1993.

Jacobs, Jeff. "Steroids Weaken Baseball Legacy." *Hartford Courant*. July 30, 2002.

Wilson, Doug. *Pudge*. New York: Thomas Dunne Books, 2015.

CHAPTER 13

Pierre Beauchamp once again came up big for me this chapter, as did CogniSens CEO Jean Castanguay, who made a great espresso.

Jeff Zimman and Greg Appelbaum also provided invaluable insight. Additional select sources:

BrainHQ.com.

BrainHQ.tb12.com.

Doraiswarmy, P. Murali, and Marc E. Agronin. "Brain Games: Do They Really Work?" *Scientific American.* April 28, 2009.

Faubert, Jocelyn. "3-D-Multiple Object Tracking training task improves passing decision-making accuracy in soccer players." *Psychology of Sport and Exercise.* June 16, 2015.

———. "Professional athletes have extraordinary skills for rapidly learning complex and neutral dynamic visual scenes." *Scientific Reports.* January 31, 2013.

Faubert, Jocelyn, and Lee Sidebottom. "Perceptual-Cognitive Training of Athletes." *Journal of Clinical Sport Psychology.* 2012.

Fitzpatrick, Richard. "How do you win the World Cup? Play Medal of Honor." *Guardian.* February 6, 2015.

Gregurić, Krešimir. "Secret training of elite soccer players." Medium.com. January 6, 2016.

Legault, Isabelle, and Jocelyn Faubert. "Perceptual-cognitive training improves biological motion perception: evidence for transferability of training in healthy aging." *Cognitive Neuroscience and Neuropsychology.* February 8, 2012.

Legault, Isabelle, et al. "Healthy older observers show equivalent perceptual-cognitive training benefits to young adults for multiple object tracking." *Frontiers in Psychology.* June 6, 2013.

Limpert, Rick. "Technology on display at NFL Combine." Examiner.com. February 25, 2012.

Mann, Derek, et al. "Perceptual-Cognitive Expertise in Sports: A Meta-Analysis." *Journal of Sport and Exercise Psychology.* 2007.

Mitroff, Sarah. "Lumosity vs. Elevate: Battle of the brain-training apps." CNET.com. August 21, 2014.

NeuroTracker.net

Parsons, Brendan, et al. "Enhancing Cognitive Function Using

Perceptual-Cognitive Training." *Clinical EEG and Neuroscience.* November 17, 2014.

PositScience.com

Sarkar, Samit. "Research shows playing first-person shooters improve learning abilities, cognitive function." *Polygon.* January 30, 2013.

Scilearn.com

Smith, Glenn E., et al. "A cognitive training program based on principles of brain plasticity: results from the Improvement in Memory with Plasticity-based Adaptive Cognitive Training (IMPACT) study." *Journal of the American Geriatrics Society.* February 9, 2009.

St. John, Allen. "Drafting a Franchise QB on NFL Draft Day? There's an App for That." *Forbes.* May 8, 2014.

Steenbergen, Laura, et al. "Action Video Gaming and Cognitive Control: Playing First Person Shooter Games Is Associated with Improved Action Cascading but Not Inhibition." *PLoS One.* December 10, 2015.

Wiltfong, Steve. "Vision training part of NFL prep." 247sports.com. February 27, 2013.

CHAPTER 14

Jason Sada at Axon Sports was another one of the very first people I spoke to about any of This Stuff, and their blog, AxonPotential.com, provided an excellent starting point for much of my research. I am very thankful.

I also very much enjoyed visiting and talking with Jason Sherwin at deCervo in New York, and Brian Miller and Wes Clapp at Neuro-Scouting in Boston.

Additional select sources:

AthletesPerformance.com.

AxonSports.com.

deCervo.com.

Myerberg, Paul. "Using technology to make college football better, faster, safer. *USA Today.* August 24, 2014.

NeuroScouting.com.

Speier, Alex. "Red Sox neuroscouting aims to find prospects' potential." *Boston Globe.* February 18, 2015.

TeamEXOS.com.

Verducci, Tom. "Moveable Beast." *Sports Illustrated.* July 1, 2015.

CHAPTER 15

Andy Walshe let me test-drive Red Bull's new F1 simulator, which was a huge rush, and I feel bad that I wrecked it.

I also learned a ton from Derek Belch at STRIVR and Brendan Reilly at EON Sports, not to mention Greg Appelbaum and David Zielinski at Duke's DiVE virtual-reality cave. That was unreal. Thanks again.

Additional select sources:

Alvarez, Edgar. "Jason Giambi bets on virtual reality to train better batters." Engadget.com. November 16, 2015.

Archer, Todd. "Cowboys to use virtual reality to help players in film study." ESPN.com. June 8, 2015.

Chen, Yu-Li. "The Effects of Virtual Reality Learning Environment on Student Cognitive and Linguistic Development." *Asia-Pacific Education Researcher.* August 2016.

Eonreality.com

Eonsportsvr.com

Feldman, Bruce. "'I was blown away': Welcome to football's quarterback revolution." FoxSports.com. March 11, 2015.

Fingas, John. "Watch the Patriots practice in VR through Google Cardboard." Engadget.com. December 6, 2015.

Graham, Peter. "Travel Inside the Game Launched by Bank of America and Visa." Vrfocus.com. December 6, 2015.

Green, Keegan. "How VR is helping train NFL quarterbacks Carson Palmer and Jameis Winston." Venturebeat.com. June 11, 2016.

King, Peter. "A Quarterback and His Game Plan, Part 1: Five Days to Learn 171 Plays." MMQB.SI.com. November 18, 2015.

Lelinwalla, Mark. "Jason Giambi Bringing Virtual Reality to Baseball Via Project OPS, an Interactive Hitting Simulator." *Tech Times.* October 22, 2015.

Medina, John. *Brain Rules.*

Multon, Frank, et al. "Using Virtual Reality to Analyze Sports Performance." *IEEE Computer Graphics and Applications.* March/April 2010.

Seymour, Neal, et al. "Virtual Reality Training Improves Operating Room Performance." *Annals of Surgery*. October 2002.

Smith, Dave. "One of the NFL's top quarterbacks trains with virtual reality." *Business Insider*. November 18, 2015.

Speier, Alex. "Red Sox neuroscouting aims to find prospects' potential." *Boston Globe*. February 18, 2015.

STRIVRLabs.com.

Tampa Bay Buccaneers. "Bucs Introduce Virtual Reality Technology." Buccaneers.com. July 20, 2015.

Tromp, Shaina. "Impact of 3-D learning in schools." CyberScience3D .com. April 9, 2015.

Yasinskas, Pat. "Bucs invest in virtual-reality system to help Jameis Winston." ESPN.com. July 20, 2015.

CHAPTER 16

Oliver Marmol, once again, was great fun to talk with and learn from, as was Brandon Payne.

Andy Walshe once again provided lots of great information, as did Jason Mihalik at the University of North Carolina–Chapel Hill, and Greg Appelbaum at Duke.

And I'm hugely grateful to Herb Yoo and Joe Bingold for having me out to their office for a day in Beaverton and letting me play with all their cool toys—and for showing me that I really did have a chance to go pro if my mind hadn't broken me. Thanks, guys.

Also, I can't forget Erez Morag, another one of the first people I talked with about This Stuff. Really wish I could have made it to Israel to see your setup, Erez. Maybe someday soon.

Additional select sources:

Acceler8.co.il.

Appelbaum, Greg, et al. "Improved visual cognition through stroboscopic training." *Frontiers in Psychology*. October 28, 2011.

Davis, Scott. "Stephen Curry does a dribbling drill with blinding glasses and a tennis ball and it looks grueling." *Business Insider*. November 6, 2016.

Holliday, Joshua. "Effect of Stroboscopic Vision Training on Dynamic Visual Acuity Scores: Nike Vapor Strobe Eyewear." Digitalcommons.usu.edu. April 2013.

Senaptec.com.

Smith, Trevor, and Stephen Mitroff. "Stroboscopic Training Enhances Anticipatory Timing." *International Journal of Exercise Science.* October 2012.

PART FOUR INTRODUCTION

Andy Walsh, Michael Gervais, and Urban Meyer were invaluable for this chapter.

Additional select sources:

Bergland, Christopher. "Holding a Grudge Produces Cortisol and Diminishes Oxytocin." *Psychology Today.* April 11, 2015.

Bettencourt, Megan Feldman. *Triumph of the Heart.* New York: Hudson Street Press, 2015.

———. "Triumph of the Heart." *Psychology Today.* June 30, 2015.

Enright, Robert, et al. "The effects of a forgiveness intervention on patients with coronary artery disease." *Taylor & Francis.* February 18, 2009.

Fox, Glenn R. "Neural correlates of gratitude." *Frontiers in Psychology.* September 30, 2015.

Hand, Douglas. "Saving Burn Victims." *New York Times Magazine.* September 15, 1985.

Martin, Sean. "USC researchers use Holocaust survivors' memories to map how brain experiences gratitude." *International Business Times.* October 20, 2015.

Sneed, Brandon. "Urban Meyer Outtake: The Strikeout." Brandon-Sneed.com. October 11, 2016.

University of Southern California. "Holocaust Survivors' Memories Help Researchers Map Brain Circuitry of Gratitude." usc.edu. No date given.

CHAPTER 17

I built most of this chapter from interviews with Andy Walshe and Pete Naschak, who spent hours talking about this and more with me. Thank you!

I also owe the Red Bull production team a big high five for their excellent documentary and footage of Acheron: Patagonia, available at RedBull.tv, as well as the excellently detailed firsthand account written by Mark Anders in the June 2013 issue of *Red Bulletin*.

CHAPTER 18

I can't thank Kyle Kingsbury enough. I interviewed him at the last possible minute, in September 2016, and rewrote this chapter to include what I learned from him. He was brave and generous to open up about his experience with ayahuasca and about his life in general. I admire him and am hugely grateful for that.

Some of my other sources for this chapter include:

Bettencourt, Megan Feldman. "Triumph of the Heart." *Psychology Today.* June 30, 2015.

Escobedo, Tricia. "Could this be the next medicinal marijuana?" CNN. October 31, 2014.

Fowlkes, Ben. "How Kyle Kingsbury used ayahuasca to become a happier person and a worse fighter." *USA Today.* August 3, 2014.

Ferris, Tim. "The Man Who Studied 1,000 Deaths to Learn How to Live." Tim Ferriss Show #153: BJ Miller. April 14, 2016.

Frood, Arran. "Ayahuasca Psychedelic Tested for Depression." *Scientific American.* April 18, 2015.

Hayes, Stephie. "Dan Hardy Gives Extremely Detailed Account of His Psychedelic Ayahuasca Experience." Bloodyelbow.com. September 15, 2012.

Morris, Bob. "Ayahuasca: A Strong Cup of Tea." *New York Times.* June 13, 2014.

Multidisciplinary Association for Psychedelic Studies. maps.org.

Salak, Kira. "Hell and Back." *National Geographic.* March 2006.

Strouder, Richard. "Veteran: My search for a PTSD cure led me to the Amazon." CNN.com. Richard Strouder. October 24, 2014.

CHAPTER 19

Crash was enormously generous with his time and facilities, spending the better part of two afternoons in Santa Monica telling me his story and letting me float around in his tanks at Float Lab. Michael Garrett was also generous, spending an hour on the phone with me from San Francisco as he told me about Reboot Spa and why he built it and how guys like Steph Curry are using it.

Some other sources I drew from to shore up my knowledge about sensory deprivation and such include:

Alipour, Sam. "Stephen Curry on copying the Warriors' way: 'You won't have the personnel.'" ESPN.com. December. 8, 2015.

Dowling, Kyle. "Time Out: The Rise of Sensory Deprivation Tanks." *Atlantic.* October 12, 2012.

Fan, Shelly. "Floating Away: The Science of Sensory Deprivation Therapy." *Discover.* April 4, 2014.

Leggett, Hadley. "Out of LSD? Just 15 Minutes of Sensory Deprivation Triggers Hallucinations." *Wired.* October 21, 2009.

Mason, O. J., and F. Brady. "The psychotomimetic effects of short-term sensory deprivation." *Journal of Nervous and Mental Disease.* October 2009.

McAleney, Patrick, et al. "Effects of Flotation Restricted Environmental Stimulation on Intercollegiate Tennis Performance." *Perceptual and Motor Skills.* 1990.

Rubin, Courtney. "Sensory Deprivation Tanks Find New Converts." *New York Times.* December 2, 2015.

Strouder, Richard. "Veteran: My search for a PTSD cure led me to the Amazon." CNN.com. October 24, 2014.

Turkewitz, Julie. "Climb In, Tune In: A Renaissance for Sensory Deprivation Tanks." *New York Times.* October 17, 2015.

EPILOGUE

One final time, I have to thank Andy Walshe for letting me hang out at Red Bull for a day. That was a blast and I learned a ton.

Also, I have to thank Michael Gervais and Urban Meyer again.

I learned some fascinating things from Elizabeth Gilbert's 2009 TED talk "Your Elusive Creative Genius," and from David Eagleman's book and PBS series, both titled *The Brain.*

Not to mention Dan Chartier and Leslie Sherlin, who showed me my brain in ways I could not believe were real, showed me how to make it better, and then showed me that it had actually gotten better. Thank you so much.

About the Author

Brandon Sneed is a writer at large for *B/R Mag* at Bleacher Report/CNN. His stories have also appeared in *Outside, ESPN The Magazine,* and more, and have twice been notable selections in *Best American Sports Writing.* He lives in Greenville, North Carolina, with his wife and son and their two dogs, a Jack Russell terrier named Cooper and a Jack Russell–pit bull mix named Jack. Sometimes when he's not writing or traveling around for research, he works out, plays softball and basketball, gets addicted to Xbox, and, every once in a while, goes for a jog. He often gets excited about other things he'd like to do, but then his body makes him sleep so his brain doesn't get more messed up than it already is.

You can keep up with him—and follow along as he tries to keep up with This Stuff and more—at BrandonSneed.com.